When the Mind Fails
A guide to dealing with incompetency

When the Mind Fails

A guide to dealing with incompetency

Michel Silberfeld ■ Arthur Fish

UNIVERSITY OF TORONTO PRESS
Toronto Buffalo London

© University of Toronto Press Incorporated 1994
Toronto Buffalo London
Printed in Canada

ISBN 0-8020-0463-6 (cloth)
ISBN 0-8020-6780-8 (paper)

Printed on acid-free paper

Canadian Cataloguing in Publication Data

Silberfeld, Michel
  When the mind fails : a guide to dealing with
  incompetency

  Includes index.
  ISBN 0-8020-0463-6 (bound)
  ISBN 0-8020-6780-8 (pbk.)

  1. Mentally ill – Care. 2. Mentally ill aged –
  Care. I. Fish, Arthur. II. Title.

  HV3004.S55 1994   362.2   C93-094593-X

Contents

Preface

This book is addressed to people who must find answers to the sometimes urgent, and always distressing, human problems that mental
incompetency often brings with it. Incompetency may afflict anyone
and its presence often arouses strong passions – anger, sorrow, and
guilt prominent among them. It engenders confusion in both the
incompetent person and those who care for him or her. Incompetency
simultaneously creates needs and impairs the ability to answer them.
It is hardly surprising, then, that incompetent people, and their relatives and friends, often seek professional assistance. Yet professional
assistance, although often indispensable, is seldom a substitute for the
thoughtful and loving care and support of relatives and friends. This
book has been written primarily for those who must struggle to understand and overcome their own feelings about incompetency, and at the
same time to understand and answer the needs of an incompetent
relative or friend. As well, it is addressed to people who fear that they
may themselves, through aging, injury, disease, or illness, become
incompetent and who wish to plan for their care and protection
should this occur. Finally, we hope the book will be of use to professionals who perform competency assessments or who must sometimes decide whether to refer a patient or client to a specialist for one.

It is often extremely difficult to decide how to care for an incompetent person. Having learned that a friend or relative is incompetent we
must come to terms with our own powerful emotions. Then would-be
caregivers must often cope with an incompetent person who is angry,
confused, disoriented, and uncooperative; contend with laws that are
inadequate or confusing; and, negotiate a health- and social-care
system whose different parts are poorly coordinated, in which there

may be no, or very few, specially trained competency assessors, and in which even well-trained and diligent professionals are often overworked and unable to devote as much time as they want to individual cases. Notwithstanding these obstacles many people maintain their desire to bestow kindness, support, and respect on their incompetent relatives and friends. The primary goal of this book is to help such people think about how they may best put their good intentions into practice.

This book's approach to incompetency is based on our experiences at the Competency Clinic at the Baycrest Centre for Geriatric Care in Toronto. The Competency Clinic is a working hospital clinic that performs competency assessments and conducts research on competency and related subjects. It was conceived by Dr Michel Silberfeld, and he is one of its three founders; he is also the coordinator who directs its daily operations. Arthur Fish is a practicing lawyer and a doctoral candidate at the University of Toronto law school; while this book was being written he was a Legal Fellow at the clinic.

What help can we, both professionals, offer to people who must struggle to deal with incompetency, day in and day out, in the varied circumstances of their own lives? Obviously, we cannot reform the laws of every American state and every Canadian province so that they provide for the protection of incompetent people in a reasonable and dignified way. Neither can we provide the financial and social resources that incompetent people often need, but lack. Yet it is possible to make too much of the difficulties that society and its institutions impose on those who provide care, and too little of what can be achieved simply by combining the will to help with some thought. Bad laws, policies, or institutions may prevent or hinder the provision of reasonable and thoughtful care, but good ones alone do not guarantee it. Indeed, the guardianship laws of our own province of Ontario are very inadequate (a problem likely soon to be remedied by new legislation), and informed commentators have argued that the laws of many American states are too. Ontario's present laws cause much frustration and a variety of problems, but still they do not prevent many people from making decent and thoughtful provision for their own or another's incompetency. The quality of the relationship between an incompetent person and his or her caregivers ultimately depends on the degree of thoughtfulness and attention that are brought to bear on it, and not on laws or institutions. Incompetency is a human problem that sometimes calls for a specialized professional response, but that always (and sometimes only) calls for a sensitive and intelligent response from those who care for incompetent people.

What this book is about

This is not a self-help book. The applicable laws, the available institutions and services, and individual needs vary widely from case to case and jurisdiction to jurisdiction, and no single book could possibly guide every reader to the best solution of his or her particular difficulties. But people often require medical and legal advice to plan for their own incompetency, or to address the needs of an incompetent person. People who are not lawyers or doctors generally should not attempt to act as either, whether on their own behalf or on behalf of another. This book does *not* offer medical or legal advice and is no substitute for seeking the advice of a doctor, lawyer, or other competent professional who is fully acquainted with the individuals whom he or she advises and with local laws, institutions, and practices. But there are some fundamental problems associated with incompetency that are both inescapable and omnipresent, and there are many similarities among the laws and social policies that apply to incompetent people in many North American jurisdictions.

In this book we discuss many commonly available legal devices or doctrines, social and health-care institutions, and medical and diagnostic procedures. For example, we frequently discuss a legal device called a power of attorney, the usefulness of which varies from country to country, state to state, and province to province, but with which all North American (and many other) lawyers should be familiar. People should not assume that in their locality a power of attorney is the appropriate legal solution to an incompetent person's problems, but they can assume that by questioning a competent lawyer about one they will sufficiently identify the kind of legal service that they wish to receive. Moreover, the book is constructed around a series of realistic, but fictional, cases and offers many concrete examples of the application of the principles of competency assessment. This is a practical, focused guide to thinking about incompetency, based on the premise that the best source of personal empowerment is knowledge and understanding. The purpose of this book is to share a specialist's knowledge with a general audience.

The Competency Clinic at the Baycrest Centre for Geriatric Care

We have already mentioned the Competency Clinic at the Baycrest Centre for Geriatric Care, and it is worthwhile to say something about the clinic's composition, work, and achievements. People increasingly recognize that an important way of protecting the liberty of vulnerable individuals without leaving them prey to their own weaknesses is to base their care on thorough and fair competency assessments. The Competency Clinic is both a model for the performance of such assessments and a forum for educating assessors. Its composition and methods are based on the principles discussed in this book, and so an introduction to the clinic is a good way to begin thinking about incompetency.

The clinic is a multidisciplinary enterprise founded on the principle that competency is not simply a medical or legal concept, but rather a complex phenomenon that has medical, social, legal, and ethical dimensions. At the time of writing the clinic's members and fellows include a psychiatrist, a psychologist, two philosophers, and two lawyers. Competency assessment as a subject of study and thought is no one's special property, and the clinic exists at the juncture of medicine, law, and philosophy; insights and knowledge drawn from all three disciplines will be found in this book.

Acknowledgments

This book, like the Competency Clinic itself, is a multidisciplinary effort. Some parts of it were obviously written by a lawyer and others by a psychiatrist. However, the approach that each of us now takes to our respective discipline has been altered by our collaboration. Indeed, our work and ideas are so intermingled that either of us could, with justification, have appeared as first author.

We have received much help and incurred many debts of gratitude while writing this book. The idea for the project was Dr Silberfeld's. Professor William Harvey of the Department of Philosophy at the University of Toronto and Professor Bernard Dickens of the Law School at the University of Toronto participated in the initial planning, as did Mr Ian Montagnes, then Assistant Director and Editor-in-Chief of the University of Toronto Press. Robert Pepper-Smith, a former Ethics Fellow at the clinic, made a substantial contribution to the material that eventually became chapters one and two. Chapter three, about the formal assessment of competency, is a record of how assessments are performed at the clinic and we acknowledge with gratitude the thoroughness, fairness, and intelligence that our colleagues Mary Finstad, Psychiatric Fellow and Lorraine Landry, Ethics Fellow brought to our collective work at the clinic, and that we have attempted to mirror in this book. A similar acknowledgment is owed to the former clinical fellows, Saara Chetner, Legal Fellow, D. Rutman, Psychiatry Fellow, and Evelyn Stein, Legal Fellow, all of whom contributed significantly to the clinic's development. We also wish to acknowledge the valuable assistance of Ann Kerwin, who performed, with diligence, enthusiasm, and skill, the thankless task of locating every relevant piece of Canadian legislation and much other valuable material. Thanks are also due to Ian Montagnes for his many valuable criticisms and suggestions and to the two anonymous reviewers who read the manuscript on behalf of University of Toronto Press. Finally, the book could not have been completed without the support of a number of institutions. We are grateful to the Laidlaw Foundation and the Law Foundation of the Law Society of Upper Canada, both of which provided grants that made it possible to write and produce the book. We are also grateful to the Ministry of Health for Ontario, the Alzheimer Society of Canada (which supports the clinic's ongoing study of substitute-decision making) and the Baycrest Centre for Geriatric Care without whose ongoing support none of the work that made the book possible could have been done. We acknowledge, of course, our sole responsibility for any errors in the book.

Both the law and the Competency Clinic's practices are described as they were in December 1991.

Michel Silberfeld and Arthur Fish

When the Mind Fails

Introduction

Incompetency has become a major social problem in large part because the number of elderly people in North America is increasing rapidly. Although incompetency afflicts people of all ages and may arise from many causes it is a problem frequently seen among the elderly. It has become increasingly evident to us, and to others, that there is a great need for a book that outlines the fundamental principles and basic practices of competency assessment. Scientific inquiry into competency is not sufficiently advanced for anyone yet to be able to write the final word on competency assessment. Moreover, there are many aspects of the Competency Clinic's work (including entire research projects) that for various reasons are not discussed in this book. However, the clinic has developed some unique methods of assessment and of working with incompetent people. These methods we think are justifiable on the basis of the scientific evidence (admittedly insufficient) that we now possess, and are also faithful to ethical and legal principles that are increasingly recognized as the proper basis for dealings with all weak and vulnerable people.

Basic principles

The increasing interest in the Competency Clinic is clearly related to increasing recognition of the ethical and legal principles on which its practices are based. Primary among these principles are:

1   The right of all competent people – including the weak, the vulnerable, and the eccentric – to make their own decisions.

2 The obligation to restrict the liberty of even clearly incompetent people only as far as it is necessary to do so for protecting them from harm.

This second obligation is sometimes referred to as the principle of the least-restrictive alternative, and it lies at the heart of this book. In essence it means this: there are usually several ways to care for or protect an incompetent person; the one to choose is the one that least restricts that person's liberty. But how does competency assessment serve these important legal and ethical principles? First, it helps distinguish those who are capable of making their own decisions (and who therefore generally have the right to do so) from those who are incapable of doing so (and who *may* therefore *sometimes* be deprived of the right to do so). Second, it pinpoints the nature and defines the extent of an individual's incompetency, and so fixes the nature and extent of the deprivation of liberty to which that person may be subjected. Competency assessment is the practical means of distinguishing those who are capable of making choices from those who are not.

Task-specific competency

The single most important concept discussed in this book is task-specific competency. Ordinarily people speak about competency as though it is a single ability that people either possess or lack. But competency is not like a light bulb that is either on or off. Rather, it is a series of abilities, some of which can be present while others are absent. People do not have competence, they have competencies. Someone may be, for example, incompetent to drive a car but quite competent to invest his or her own money. Or, a person may be competent to consent to one medical treatment (say, stitching a wound) but incapable of consenting to another (say, brain surgery). Competency must be measured in relation to specific acts that people wish to perform or consent to. The assessment of competency in relation to specific tasks is sometimes called 'functional assessment.'

   The best modern guardianship legislation (for example, the laws of Florida and Michigan in the United States and of Alberta in Canada) requires or encourages task-specific assessments and tailors a guardian's powers to correspond as closely as possible to the incompetent person's disabilities. For example, a guardian might be allowed to make financial decisions on a person's behalf but not decisions about the person's medical treatment. Even in the absence of such guardianship legislation, however, competency assessors bear an important responsibility to guard peoples' liberty. Unfortunately, assessors (and many others who deal with failing or vulnerable individuals) do not always recognize the degree or nature of this responsibility. Too often they think that the zealous protection of liberty is incompatible with the provision of respectful, thoughtful, and decent care. Indeed, there are times when liberty and well-being conflict, but competency assessment is a means of avoiding or mediating such conflicts. Thorough and careful assessments not only distinguish incompetency from competency, but they may also identify means of overcoming disabilities or of tailoring care so that it restricts liberty as little as possible. Respect for a person's liberty is an integral part of caring for him or her, and competency assessment is the practical means of integrating liberty and care.

Competency and capacity

In this book we generally use the word competency to describe the mental ability to perform a particular task or tasks. In some contexts, especially when discussing the law, we also use the word 'capacity.' In general, the two words are synonymous. However, there is a reason why the law increasingly tends to use the word capacity in preference to competency. Too often in the past people have viewed competency assessment as akin to an examination for a driver's license. To be a good driver one must perform set tasks – parallel parking, driving in reverse, etc. – with a certain degree of proficiency. To be mentally competent, it was thought similarly, a person must perform other kinds of set tasks with a certain degree of proficiency. The problem with this approach is that not all activities are like driving. It is reasonable to require all drivers to meet a common standard of proficiency, but it is not reasonable to impose a common standard on every area of human conduct. For example, some people value money highly, and others do not. People who value money highly will tend to set a very high standard for diligence and precision in the conduct of their personal finances; conversely, people who do not value money highly may set a low standard of care in the conduct of their finances. A person who is sloppy about finances is not necessarily incompetent, but if judged by the 'driver's examination' approach to competency might be found to be so. That approach imposes conventional expectations and choices on all people. In reaction, modern laws tend to use the word 'capacity' as a signal that those who assess competency should focus on abilities to make and execute choices, rather than on the wisdom or folly of the choices that are made. This book endorses this approach to assessment, and demonstrates its implementation.

In practice, however, the legal test for mental competency is sometimes explained in a way that invites confusion. Lawyers sometimes say that competency or capacity must be judged, as far as possible, by people's innate abilities rather than by their actions. This formulation is misleading, because there is an indissoluble connection between capacity and actions. Competency and incompetency are not abstract entities; rather they are complex assemblies of abilities and disabilities that manifest themselves as success or failure in the conduct of activities. There is no magic device that permits us to peer inside people and determine what facilities or 'capacity' they possess. Thus, capacity is generally best assessed by looking at what people actually do in the circumstances of their own lives. The essential issue is not to avoid judging a person's conduct, but rather to avoid judging it according to a conventional standard of competence as opposed to that individual's own habitual or considered decisions and values.

The law

Although there are common themes among the North American laws that govern decision making on behalf of incompetent people (that is, substitute decision making) there are also many differences of detail. For example, some form of court-appointed guardianship is available virtually everywhere in North America (and in many other parts of the world as well), but the nature and degree of incompetency sufficient to justify a guardianship order, the kind of assessment required to obtain it, and the guardian's powers, all vary from place to place. Only a legal textbook could provide accurate information about the laws that apply to incompetent people and substitute decision making in each North American province, state, district, and territory, and this book is not a legal textbook. Rather it identifies situations in which people commonly require legal advice and offers some very general information about legal devices (like durable powers of attorney, guardianship, and wills) that are widely used to meet the needs of incompetent people. It is intended to give its readers the tools to identify a proper answer to an incompetent person's needs, or to plan for their own care and protection if they should become incompetent. Thus, it is filled with examples of how the law, and legal planning, affect competency assessment. In every case an attempt is made to illustrate general principles and approaches with laws or legal doctrines that, although drawn from a particular province or state, are typical of their kind and so widely relevant.

The general approach that this book takes to the law – which is to emphasize legal devices that maximize the ability of people to make their own decisions – is certainly applicable everywhere. But the specific means of implementing this general goal will vary from person to person, and from jurisdiction to jurisdiction, because both individuals' needs and local laws differ. Readers should not take any legal information or doctrine that is discussed in this book as advice that applies directly to their own lives or to the lives of their incompetent relatives or friends.

CHAPTER ONE

What is incompetency?

When talking about competency and incompetency we are dealing with matters that lie close to the core of our humanity. The word competent literally means 'having sufficient ability' to perform a specific task, and it is related to a number of other terms, like independence, self-esteem, and happiness, that are commonly used to describe the qualities of a life that is worth living. Competency is a person's ability to make, and act on, his or her own decisions. The ability to decide what to do, and then to do it, is closely connected with how people feel and think about themselves and how others think and feel about them: a person's competency, in large measure, is what he or she is.

Denying that another person is competent challenges the foundation of that person's independence and dignity. It is wrong to question lightly another's mental competency: the challenge will certainly cause pain and may do even worse harm. But this raises a conflict for which there probably is no completely satisfactory resolution. People sometimes insist on doing something that they are incompetent to do (like driving a car although their eyesight is failing) and thereby present a real threat of harm to themselves and others. Then it may be necessary to challenge another's competence (for example, by writing a letter to the Ministry of Transport saying that the person's licence to drive should be revoked for incompetence). Yet if people are permitted to challenge one another's competence there is inevitably a risk that they will do so improperly. We may treat someone as incompetent who really is not, or (and this is a very common mistake) we may exaggerate the degree of the other person's incompetency and force more help on that person than he or she either needs or wants. The problem is to recognize two obligations simultaneously – on the one hand, the obligation to assist incompetent people who require help and, on the other, the obligation to respect the liberty of people, including the right of incompetent people to make those decisions that they *are* competent to make.

In practice, the potential conflict between care and liberty can be resolved by assessing competency in relation to the person's own habits and choices. The starting point is to make the assessment in relation to a specific task or aspect of life, to consider what the person wants to achieve for himself or herself in that connection, and then to ask what abilities that person needs to succeed on his or her own terms. For example, consider an assessment of financial competency that is focused on a person's ability to do his personal banking. The initial question commonly should be: 'What does it mean to say that this person is competent to conduct his own banking?' The answer will vary according to how much the person values money, how much money he or she has, and what he or she wishes or needs to do with it. Having answered the question the assessor would then generate a list of criteria for the successful conduct of the person's banking. The individualization of a competency assessment to take account of personal preferences, decisions, and wishes, may seem to be, but is not, a daunting task. Questions about competency tend to arise in respect of the same matters – most frequently, finances and medical care – and many problems and issues arise repeatedly in competency assessments. Thus, when financial competency is in issue it is very common for assessors to consider the allegedly incompetent person's ability to do his or her own banking. A good way to begin thinking about competency, then, is to consider some very common problems that are reflected in the following nine fictional case histories.

These nine cases are typical of the circumstances in which competency often becomes an issue. They also introduce the social, medical, and legal frameworks within which competency assessments are made virtually everywhere in North America. Further, they illustrate two important points. One, competency issues arise in the context of daily life, so that judgments of competency (albeit informal and subject to revision) can be made well by anyone who is prepared to think about how people perform the basic tasks involved in the management of their own lives. Two, and more important, in the real world it is not possible to separate the assessment of competency from the intense, and often conflicting, emotions that we feel when our competency is called into question, or when we challenge another's competency. It is essential to remember that allegations of incompetency are often advanced by, and in respect of, human beings who are struggling to cope with the unhappy consequences of aging, illness, or brain injury.

Choosing one's residence

Every competent adult has the right to decide where and with whom he or she will live. But there are times when people are incapable of recognizing that they are likely to harm themselves, or others, if they do not live in a supervised or controlled environment. It sometimes is necessary to deprive people of the right to decide where they will live. In most parts of North America there are three common ways in which incompetent people may lawfully be deprived of the right to choose their own residence.

1   A court can appoint a guardian who has the power to make personal decisions, including choice of residence, for a person who is incapable of making his or her own. Guardians are identified by different names in different parts of North America (these names include guardian, committee, conservator, curator, and fiduciary), but they serve the same function everywhere; guardians have the legal power and duty to care for the person, or the property, or both, of someone who is mentally incapable of doing for himself or herself.

2   A person (who may be called a creator, grantor, donor, or principal, depending on the laws or practices of particular jurisdictions) may, in anticipation of incompetency, execute a document called an enduring or durable power of attorney which gives another person (who may be called a donee, grantee, agent, attorney, or attorney-in-fact) the right to make decisions for the principal should he or she become incapable of making his or her own. In some places the law explicitly permits people to empower an attorney to make decisions about residence. In others the attorney in effect has this power because he or she has the right to decide, for example, whether an incompetent person's home should be kept or sold.

3   People may be involuntarily institutionalized under mental-health laws. This process is sometimes called 'civil commitment' or 'invol-

untary hospitalization,' and in many North American jurisdictions is available only if a person suffers from a mental illness as a result of which he or she is (or is likely to be) dangerous to himself or herself or to others, or suffers from a mental illness as a result of which he or she is under a grave disability in providing for his or her basic personal needs. Civil commitment may not be applicable to every person who is incompetent to make decisions about his or her place of residence. Moreover, even where civil commitment is available it is often a poor answer to an incompetent person's needs, and it is especially unsuitable for elderly people.

The issue of capacity to choose one's residence is often raised when a person is in hospital for the treatment of an illness and will soon be ready to be discharged. In assessing the competency of such people it is often necessary to consider both their ability to choose the place where they will live (choice of residence) and their ability to function in the place they have chosen (ability to thrive). Although these two kinds of competency are conceptually distinct, in practice they are often connected; in this book they are considered together. However the power to make decisions about where a person will live is obtained, it should be exercised only in cases of absolute necessity, for determining the circumstances of one's daily existence is almost a definition of what it means to be, and to be accepted as, an adult person.

Case 1: Alzheimer's disease

Mr L.H. is an elderly widower who, four years ago, following the death of his wife of forty-two years, went to live with his daughter and her husband (the children). Two years ago Mr L.H. started to become forgetful. The first indication of his deteriorating memory was his misplacing things and becoming panic stricken when he could not find them. He became extremely suspicious of the children and began to accuse them of stealing the things that he had misplaced himself. He also began to tell people that his children were plotting to harm him. The children recognized that Mr L.H. was suffering from some kind of serious problem, and they sought the help of their family physician. She examined Mr L.H. and referred him to a neurologist (a medical doctor who specializes in disorders of the nervous system and brain). The neurologist's diagnosis was that Mr L.H. was in the early stages of a progressive dementia, most likely Alzheimer's disease. 'Dementia' is a term used to describe a number of mental disorders that are marked by the loss of short- and long-term memory, impaired thinking and judgment, disturbances in other mental functions (like speech), or marked changes in personality. A progressive dementia, of which Alzheimer's disease is probably the best known, is one that will inevitably continue to worsen. Dementia is a very common cause of incompetence in the elderly.

Mr L.H.'s daughter is in her early fifties and has three children, two of whom attend university and require substantial financial support from their parents. Her husband is a construction foreman, whose work often requires him to be away from home for long periods. Even when he is not travelling, he works very long days and returns home too exhausted to provide much help with Mr L.H.'s care. The family has a comfortable income, but they cannot afford to pay anyone to assist in caring for Mr L.H., so the burden of caring for him falls entirely on his daughter. Although he has been informed by the neurologist of his diagnosis Mr L.H. refuses to accept it, and he denies that there is anything wrong with him. His daughter knows that he will eventually deteriorate to the point where he requires assistance of a kind that she cannot possibly provide, but she refuses to consider placing her father in a nursing home or similar facility.

During the past six months Mr L.H.'s condition has deteriorated to the point where he requires virtually constant attention. He cannot control his bladder, and his bowel control is poor; although he frequently soils his clothing and the furniture (leaving his daughter to clean the resulting mess), he refuses to wear diapers, which is the only possible way of alleviating the problem. He bathes irregularly and refuses to accept help in the bath although he is incapable of managing alone (he recently left the water running in the bathtub, causing considerable water damage to the house). He spills food at every meal. He is increasingly given to fits of panic or irrational anger. Mr L.H.'s son-in-law recently raised with Mr L.H. the possibility of his moving permanently to a nursing home, or accepting periodic, temporary stays in hospital (this is known as respite care, because the patient is admitted to hospital solely to give the person looking after him or her a break or 'respite'). Mr L.H. became extremely angry when these suggestions were presented to him and refused to consider either. In fact, the attempt to discuss his care with Mr L.H. resulted only in a marked increase in his anger and suspiciousness; he now complains to anyone who will listen that his son-in-law and daughter want to 'throw him out' so that they can take all his money. A recent incident, during which Mr L.H. fled in a panic to a neighbor's home and pleaded for protection from his daughter, who (he told the neighbor) was stealing money from him, pushed his daughter to the breaking point. The family's physician has advised the husband that his wife is on the edge of collapse and that he must relieve her somehow of the burden of caring for her father.

The wife is clearly in no emotional state to realistically assess how she may best answer her father's needs without exceeding her own limits. In consultation with the physician the husband decides that the only realistic option is for Mr L.H. to move to a nursing home. Knowing that Mr L.H. is adamantly opposed to such a move the physician advises the husband that Mr L.H. can be moved to a nursing home against his will only if the children are willing to become his court-appointed guardians and that the first step toward becoming a guardian is to have Mr L.H.'s mental competency assessed. Different laws require or permit different kinds of professionals to perform assessments. In the past the laws tended to permit assessments to be performed only by medical doctors, but modern laws tend to broaden the range of permissible assessors to include psychologists and social workers. The physician agrees to refer Mr L.H. to a psychiatrist who performs competency assessments.

Case 2: A medical emergency

Mrs R.H., an elderly widow who has lived alone for many years, was hospitalized with a broken hip suffered when she slipped on ice outside her apartment building. She has received therapy in the hospital and has recovered much of her physical mobility, but she is forgetful and disoriented; occasionally she must be prompted to attend to her personal needs (like bathing), and she sometimes appears to think that she is in her apartment rather than the hospital. Her ability to perform essential personal activities, like cooking, has been assessed by an occupational therapist (often called an OT) who works in the hospital. (An OT is a health-care professional who specializes in assessing mental and physical disabilities that hinder people in the performance of tasks – particularly those essential for daily living, like washing and cooking – and in devising ways to overcome them.) The OT found that Mrs R.H. had great difficulty using an iron to press her clothes and neglected to disconnect the iron when she finished with it; she was also very clumsy when using the stove burner and spilled the contents of a pan on the open fire. The OT concluded that Mrs R.H. is at risk of setting a fire if she lives alone. A nurse reports that on at least one occasion in the hospital Mrs R.H. almost fell while adjusting the water faucets in the shower. Mrs R.H. appears to need daily assistance from a nurse or housekeeper if she is to live alone, but she can neither afford to pay anyone to assist her nor does she qualify for public assistance in this regard.

Fearing, on the basis of the OT's and the nurse's reports, that if Mrs R.H. returns home alone she will be at considerable risk of falling, or of setting a fire, her physician recommends that she move to a nursing home. Mrs R.H. denies that she is at substantial risk of falling or setting a fire. She admits that she will face more risks to her safety in her own home than she will in a nursing home, but she is prepared to run those risks. She demands to return home. He physician, the OT, and the nurse who witnessed the near-fall in the shower, all think that Mrs R.H. is incompetent to decide where she will live. Their opinion is that she does not really understand the risks she will face living at home alone, and they have informally investigated the possibility of asking the public trustee to apply to become her personal guardian. The public trustee (also sometimes called the public curator or guardian) is a public official who has the legal authority to intervene in the lives of incompetent people who are in need of assistance.

Case 3: Health care and residence

Ms M.R. is in her early fifties. She is a diabetic, and was recently hospitalized following a stroke. She was quite confused and disoriented when first admitted to hospital, but she has improved quite considerably since then. She knows that she is in the hospital, that she has suffered a stroke, and that she is exposed to a great risk of harm if she does not eat a proper diet and use her insulin properly. She is anxious to return to her home, but her physicians think that she is incompetent to make this decision because she does not appreciate the extent to which her stroke has deprived her of the abilities (particularly reliable short-term memory and adequate concentration) that in the past allowed her to attend to her own needs. Her diabetes is quite severe, and it does not take much of a deviation from her routine to create a serious risk to her health and life; if she fails to take her insulin as required, or takes the wrong amount, or eats the wrong foods, or even the right foods at the wrong time or in the wrong amounts, her blood sugar will plummet and she will likely go into shock. In effect Ms M.R.'s physicians are saying that her choice of residence is a health-care decision and that if she fully appreciated the nature of her illness, and the affect of her stroke on her ability to care for herself, she would willingly remain in a hospital or some other supervised environment where care would be administered to her. They therefore ask a hospital psychiatrist who has specialized training in competency assessment (and who leads a competency assessment team composed of himself, a medical ethicist, a nurse, and a social worker) to assess Ms M.R. If she is found to be incompetent her physicians intend to ask her family to apply to a court to become her guardian with the power to decide where she should live.

Making a will

All competent adults have the right to decide who will have their property after they die (subject to obligations to their creditors and dependents). Unfortunately, people who suffer from mental illness, mental handicap, or brain injury, and even some people who are simply old and frail, are sometimes unable to appreciate the effect of making a will or changing an existing one. If such people make wills they sometimes run a very substantial risk of being abused by unscrupulous people or of inadvertently harming those whom they would, if competent, wish to benefit. The law therefore imposes a special test of mental competency on everyone who makes a will or who alters an existing one. Testators must have what is called 'testamentary capacity,' that is, the ability to assess what they have, to recognize all those who might have a valid claim on their benevolence, and to make an independent decision about what, or how much, they will leave to whom.

The person who makes a will is usually called a 'testator'; a female testator is sometimes called a 'testatrix,' but in this book both male and female will-makers are described as testators. The person who takes charge of someone's property after he or she dies, and who follows the directions in the will, is called an 'executor'; a female executor is sometimes called an 'executrix,' but in this book both male and female estate managers are called executors. A gift made in a will is called a 'bequest,' and the person who receives the gift is generally called a 'beneficiary' (although the term 'legatee' is sometimes also used).

Case 4: Disinheriting thoughtless relatives

Late in her eighties Mrs W. suffered a stroke that impaired her memory and left her prone to confusion. She was in hospital for several months after her stroke, and then she moved to a nursing home where she now lives. In the mornings she is quite alert and fairly clear in her thinking; toward evening she becomes confused and has difficulty finding her room or recognizing people. She tells her oldest son, who is her executor, that she wants to change her existing will. She is very upset at several of the people (all of them relatives) to whom she has left a bequest in her existing will. She had originally considered them very good friends, but they have either never, or seldom, visited her in the nursing home although they could do so without much difficulty; she therefore wishes to cut them out of her will and to leave more to those family members (including her oldest son) who visit her often and who help her in many ways, sometimes with great inconvenience to themselves. Although she is sometimes forgetful about other matters, Mrs W. is insistent about wanting to change her will and repeatedly raises the issue until her son arranges for her to consult with her lawyer.

Mrs W.'s lawyer fears that she lacks testamentary capacity because she cannot recall the contents of her existing will and because her level of alertness and clarity of thought fluctuate. Moreover, he thinks it is quite likely that the family members Mrs W. wishes to disinherit will later challenge any new will that she makes, claiming that she lacked testamentary capacity or that her son exercised an 'undue influence' over her decision. The lawyer says that common sense, the law, and professional ethics and experience forbid him from helping Mrs W. make a new will without first being assured by a qualified specialist that she has testamentary capacity. Mrs W.'s son therefore approaches the medical director of the nursing home, who arranges to have a psychologist who is experienced in assessing the competency of the elderly visit her to assess her testamentary capacity. (A psychologist is a health-care professional who has received professional training and accreditation in matters relating to human thought, sensation, and behavior. Clinical psychologists who actually work with patients – like the person who will assess Mrs W. – usually hold a graduate-level degree, and, in many places, are subject to laws and a professional regulatory body similar to those that control the activities of physicians.)

Financial decisions

Competent adults have the right, subject to their obligations to support their spouses and dependents and to pay their lawful debts, to dispose of their property as they wish. But sometimes mental illnesses, handicaps, or brain injuries deprive people of the ability to conduct their own financial affairs, and they make bad decisions that cause them needless distress; such people may even inadvertently impoverish themselves or their families. Moreover, incompetent people are often easy targets for financial abuse, ranging from family pressure to spend money for others' benefit to outright theft. It is necessary to deprive some people of the control of their own financial affairs.

Everywhere in North America there are legal mechanisms by which people may, for their own protection, be deprived of control (or deprive themselves of control) over their own property or finances. One such mechanism is the judicial appointment of a guardian who has the authority to make financial decisions for a person incapable of making her or his own. Another common mechanism of substitute financial decision making is an enduring power of attorney that permits an attorney to assume control of his or her principal's finances or property if a particular contingency occurs (for example, if the principal is certified as financially incompetent by two named assessors). In many cases loss of control over one's finances is precipitated by a medical crisis of some kind; indeed, illness often does deprive people, especially older people, of the ability to manage (either mentally or physically, or both) their own financial affairs. However, medical crises, like other kinds of crisis, sometimes abate. A common problem, illustrated by the following case, is that, once someone has been hospitalized and assessed as financially incompetent, others are later unduly reluctant to accept that the person has recovered his or her financial competence.

Case 5: Financial decisions

Mr F.C., a wealthy investor whose property includes some valuable buildings and a substantial portfolio of stocks and bonds, recently suffered a stroke that left him with permanent brain damage. He was originally aphasic (aphasia means a disorder of speech, in this case an almost complete inability to talk) and partially paralyzed on the right side of his body. His speech was limited to a few phrases of two or three words in length (for example, he could say 'not now') that sometimes were sufficient to allow him to express assent to or disapproval of others' suggestions, but that were insufficient to allow him to express directly his own desires and thoughts. His difficulties in communicating were compounded by the almost complete paralysis of his right hand, which prevented him from writing. The management of Mr F.C.'s financial affairs became an urgent concern: his properties required ongoing supervision and repair, but no one had the legal authority to do either. In his investment portfolio were some stocks that he had intended to hold for only a short period and that were rapidly declining in value and bonds that had matured and were no longer earning interest. If someone capable did not soon obtain the authority to manage Mr F.C.'s properties and make investment decisions on his behalf he would likely suffer financial losses, and perhaps very severe ones.

Mr F.C. and his wife love one another, but they have always fought about money matters; he often tells her that she lacks any business sense or financial acumen. The wife informs the physician of the urgent need for her to take control of her husband's finances; she does not tell him that her husband has never trusted her financial judgment. Mr F.C. was very confused for several months after the accident, but his confusion had substantially cleared by the time the issue of financial management became pressing. He was able to move freely about the convalescent hospital where he lived, and although he could not read (there were indications that he would eventually be able to) he followed conversations, movies, and television programs closely, and his facial and gestural responses to them were appropriate and strongly indicative of comprehension and understanding.

His physician concluded that Mr F.C.'s inability to speak or read had made it impossible for him to manage his financial affairs. The physician saw that Mr and Mrs F.C. had a close and loving relationship, and Mrs F.C. seemed to the physician to be an intelligent, capable, and honest person whose primary concern was the protection of her husband's well-being. Quite naturally, the physician assumed that Mrs F.C. would be her husband's first choice to take control of his property and investments. Aware of the urgent need for some-one to take charge of the finances, the physician suggested to Mr F.C. that his wife might wish to consult a lawyer about obtaining the legal authority to manage his affairs. Much to the physician's surprise, Mr F.C. became visibly upset at this suggestion, and remained so for several days. Mr F.C.'s heated, and seemingly irrational, response to an apparently reasonable suggestion caused the physician to reconsider Mr F.C.'s competency and to conclude that not only was Mr F.C. incompetent to manage his financial affairs but that he was also incapable of selecting someone to act on his behalf. The physician thus concluded that he had no alternative to certifying Mr F.C. as financially incompetent, so that the public trustee would take over his affairs. He was surprised when Mr F.C., whom he had expected to react badly to his decision, appeared to welcome it. To the doctor this strange reaction seemed further proof of Mr F.C.'s incompetence.

Over the year following his financial certification Mr F.C. has staged a remarkable recovery. Although he is easily fatigued, he can speak with suffi-cient fluency to communicate most of his desires. He is able to make decisions for himself, but his memory has been permanently impaired. He will soon be discharged from the hospital, and he wishes to regain control of his property from the public trustee. He asks his physician to cancel the certificate of financial incompetence and to report to the public trustee that he (that is, Mr F.C.) is now capable of managing his own affairs, but the physician refuses to do either. Mrs F.C. has repeatedly told the physician that she believes her husband to be financially incompetent. When she learns that her husband wishes to take control of his property she tells the physician that she will sue him if he declares her husband to be financially competent and Mr F.C. subsequently makes financial decisions that result in losses. Uncertain of the nature and extent of his own legal obligations, fearful of a lawsuit, and having already been caught once between husband and wife (Mr F.C. has explained to him why he preferred to have the public trustee and not Mrs F.C. oversee his financial affairs), the physician decides to turn the problem over to an expert and refers Mr F.C. to a psychiatrist for an assessment of his financial competency.

Case 6: Head injury

Mr N.C. is in his late twenties. Five years ago he was struck by a car while riding his motorcycle. The accident left him a paraplegic and initially deprived him of the abilities to read, write, or speak. The accident was the fault of the car's driver, who was drunk at the time. Mr N.C.'s parents have successfully sued the car's driver on Mr N.C.'s behalf, and he will soon receive a substantial amount of money from the driver's insurance company. Mr N.C. will almost certainly never be able to earn enough money to purchase the special equipment, such as a car with hand controls or a kitchen outfitted to accommodate a person in a wheelchair, that he needs if he is to live a relatively independent life; indeed, it is an open question whether he will never be able to sustain paid employment. In short, Mr N.C.'s independence and happiness depend on the careful management of the money from the legal action.

Mr N.C. has worked very hard to regain as much physical mobility, and as many mental skills, as he can; he has, for example, learned anew how to read, write, and speak – abilities that his physicians thought he was unlikely ever to regain. His parents are his court-appointed guardians. He frequently disagrees with decisions that they make on his behalf and thinks that they have not recognized the extent of his recovery. A heated dispute has arisen between Mr N.C. and his parents over his future accommodation. Mr N.C. currently resides in a chronic-care hospital that he will soon be able to leave. Some of the money from the lawsuit will be used to build him a home of his own, equipped to accommodate his physical disabilities. His parents want the home to be located near their own suburban home, arguing that he will often need their help and advice. Mr N.C. wishes to live in the downtown area of the city so that he will be close to his friends, to entertainment, and to an active street-life; he argues that he will be able to hire people to help attend to his physical needs (for example, to do his shopping for him), that he can seek his parents' help and advice by telephone, and that he will ultimately learn to drive so that he can visit them. Although he does not say so to his parents, Mr N.C.'s primary concern is that if he lives close to them his life and decisions will be under constant parental scrutiny and criticism. Mr N.C. has also told his parents that he wishes to make more financial decisions for himself, but they refuse to allow him to do so. He intends to bring a judicial application to remove the guardianship order and asks a psychiatrist who works at the chronic-care hospital to assess his financial competency.

Health-care decisions

Competent adults everywhere in North America have the right to accept or reject medical treatment. A physician who wishes to treat a competent person must ordinarily first obtain his or her consent. A physician who wishes to treat an incompetent patient must ordinarily seek a substitute consent, usually from a spouse or relative, before administering the treatment. The term 'substitute consent,' as used in this book, incorporates two distinct but related phenomena. The first is a situation where someone merely expresses or implements a decision that someone now incapable made while competent. The second is a situation where someone actually makes a decision on behalf of an incapable person whose own wishes regarding the proposed treatment are unknown. But why allow, for example, a family member who has little knowledge of medicine to make a medical decision while denying that right to a physician who is a medical expert? There are at least two important reasons for allowing a substitute decision maker who has no medical training to make a decision that a physician cannot. First, it is generally a good idea to require physicians to explain and justify their decisions to a third party who knows the patient. For example, that person may decide that a second opinion is called or, or that the physician is unaware of relevant information, such as the patient's allergy to antibiotics or anaesthesia. Second, and more important, decisions about medical treatment often need to be made in the light of personal circumstances as well as medical criteria. A friend or relative is likely to have a better knowledge than the physician has of the person, and so a better ability to make a decision that either approximates what the person's own would be or that is in the person's best interest.

Many states and some provinces now have legislation that permits people to make what are known as 'living wills' that specify the kind of treatment that they wish to receive, or not to receive, if they are terminally ill and incompetent to make their own decisions. Often the legislation also permits people to name someone who will either implement their decisions for them or make decisions about matters not explicitly addressed in the living will. As well, many states and some provinces recognize legal devices (commonly known as durable powers of attorney for health care, health-care powers of attorney, or health-care proxies) by which people choose or instruct the substitute decider who will make medical decisions for them if they become incompetent to make their own decisions. Court-appointed guardians of the person can also sometimes make health-care decisions for incompetent people, although the extent of this power varies from jurisdiction to jurisdiction in North America. Finally, in very difficult cases, either a public official or a court may be asked to make treatment decisions for an incompetent person or to resolve doubts about who has the right to decide and on what basis. In the United States the *Quinlan* and *Cruzan* cases are well-known examples of such judicial decision making. In Canada the decision in the case of *Eve*, a young retarded woman whose mother wished to have her sterilized, is less well known but another example of judicial intervention to protect the rights of an incompetent person.

Case 7: End-of-life care

Ms C.S. is in the terminal stage of multiple sclerosis, a disease from which she has suffered for two decades. She can no longer walk, speak, or write, and she is losing her ability to swallow. Her comprehension and understanding, however, appear to be intact. She is attentive when people speak to her, and her facial expressions display her enjoyment of conversation and social events. She regularly attends gatherings in the chronic-care hospital where she lives, and appears to receive great pleasure from listening to music. Ms C.S. is losing weight rapidly because of her difficulty swallowing, and she will soon die from lack of nutrition unless a feeding tube, through which nutrition can be sent directly to her stomach without her having to chew or swallow, is inserted. The insertion of a feeding tube is a relatively minor medical procedure that carries little risk of harm to her, although the tube or the process of tube feeding may later cause discomfort or other difficulties. Ms C.S.'s life expectancy is quite short whether she receives the tube or not, but the decision about the feeding tube will determine the conditions of her dying. She has no relatives who can give or refuse a substitute consent on her behalf, and her inability to speak has so far prevented her from expressing her own wishes. The physician thinks that Ms C.S. probably has the mental ability to make her own decision about a feeding tube, and he very much wants to give her the opportunity to make up her own mind and express her own wishes about receiving one. However, given the extent of Ms C.S.'s impairment the physician can think of no way to communicate with her about such a sensitive and complex matter as her wishes regarding end-of-life treatment. The physician therefore enlists the help of both the hospital's psychiatrist and a speech therapist.

A speech therapist (also known as a speech pathologist or, more formally, as a speech-language pathologist) is a health-care professional who diagnoses and helps people overcome their problems with speech, language, and swallowing. Speech pathologists frequently work with brain-injured people and so are trained to recognize various kinds of mental disabilities that impair understanding or communication and so, too, competency. Speech therapists often become involved with cases like that of Ms C.S. where reliable communication must be established before the issue of competency can be addressed. In other cases speech therapists may help decide whether an individual's problem is mental incompetency or an inability to express himself or herself. Finally, speech therapists work as an integral part of the treatment team in many health-care institutions and especially in chronic-care hospitals. Often speech therapists have spent a great deal of time with their patients and are familiar with their needs and wishes; such information is often valuable in a competency assessment. Indeed, the speech therapist whose assistance is enlisted in Ms C.S.'s case has already worked with her for swallowing problems and knows her very well.

Powers of attorney

A power of attorney is a legal document by which one person (in this book usually called the 'principal') appoints another (in this book usually called the 'attorney') to make or execute decisions on the principal's behalf. Powers of attorney are most often used to give someone (or some group) of people full or partial control of another's financial affairs, although they can, in some provinces and states, be used as well for other purposes (primarily to appoint a substitute decision maker to make health-care decisions). The act of creating a power of attorney is called 'granting' or 'executing' it. Traditionally, a power of attorney became invalid when its maker became mentally incompetent to make his or her own decisions. In most North American jurisdictions (especially in the United States) this is no longer the law, and a power of attorney may remain valid notwithstanding the mental incompetency of its maker. A power of attorney that remains valid after the donor becomes incompetent is often called an 'enduring' or 'durable' power of attorney; a durable power of attorney that applies to medical or other personal-care decisions is often called a 'durable power of attorney for health care.'

Case 8: A good plan made too late

Mr P.A. suffers from a progressive dementia that is very rare and difficult to diagnose; but his illness is now quite advanced and therefore more easily recognized. In the early stages of his illness, before anyone knew that he had a progressive dementia, Mr P.A. became extremely moody and quixotic, unpredictably and unreasonably lashing out verbally at his wife and children; he also began to spend large amounts of money recklessly. To protect her family from financial ruin Mrs P.A. prevented Mr P.A. from writing checks or making major purchases. Ultimately, she forced him to move out of the family home because she believed that his improvident spending was evidence of an extramarital affair. She told Mr P.A. that she would not allow him back into their home unless he sought help, by which she meant help in coming to terms with his unfaithfulness and avoiding any repetition of it. Mr P.A. met with a psychiatrist who recognized the symptoms of dementia in him and who referred him to a neurologist. The neurologist diagnosed Mr P.A.'s disease and explained to Mrs P.A. that her husband's unusual behavior was caused by illness and was entirely beyond his control. The neurologist said that Mr P.A.'s condition was unstable and would certainly continue to deteriorate. She told Mr and Mrs P.A. that they should make arrangements for someone to take charge of Mr P.A.'s financial affairs, and that other people in Mr P.A.'s situation often execute a power of attorney giving someone, usually their spouses, the legal authority to make decisions for them. Mr P.A. said that he wanted Mrs P.A. to take charge of his finances and that he would like to sign a power of attorney. Neither the neurologist nor Mrs P.A. was certain, however, whether Mr P.A. really understood what a power of attorney was. They agreed that Mr and Mrs P.A. would consult with a lawyer and that the neurologist would refer Mr P.A. to a psychiatrist specializing in competency assessment.

Instructing a lawyer

In many instances a person who wishes to assert his or her legal rights requires a lawyer's assistance. A lawyer, like a doctor, can act only with the client's consent. This means that a lawyer, again like a doctor, cannot generally act on the instructions of a person who is mentally incompetent to give them (that is, who cannot understand the nature or likely consequences of the instructions that he or she issues). Thus, for example, lawyers have a duty not to bring lawsuits on the instruction of people who neither can appreciate what a lawsuit is nor are capable of participating in its conduct. But just as there are substitute deciders who make health-care decisions for incompetent people there are substitute deciders who can make legal decisions for them. In some cases a court-appointed guardian of person or property, or an attorney under an enduring power of attorney, may have the authority to make substitute legal decisions. As well, in many places the law provides for a limited form of guardianship that relates specifically to the conduct of legal cases. This limited guardian is called, depending on local laws and practices, an incompetent person's 'litigation guardian,' 'next friend,' or 'guardian *ad litem.*' Whatever the name, the function is the same everywhere in North America – namely, to accept the responsibility of instructing a lawyer on the preparation and conduct of litigation that is brought on behalf of (or against) an incompetent person.

Case 9: A marital dispute

Mrs N.L. has suffered for many years from a severe mental illness called schizophrenia that periodically renders her psychotic. Psychosis (as defined by the American Psychiatric Association) often deprives people of the ability to correctly evaluate 'the accuracy of [their] perceptions and thoughts and [likely to make] incorrect inferences about external reality, even in the face of contrary evidence.' Mrs N.L. has been held as an involuntary patient in a psychiatric hospital on several occasions, each time suffering from delusions that the Royal Canadian Mounted Police were plotting with her parents to kill her and that they were controlling her thoughts by transmitting radio waves directly to her brain. Now that she regularly takes an antipsychotic drug, and with the ongoing but infrequent assistance of a psychiatrist, her disease is relatively stable; she does not usually suffer from delusions, and those she does experience generally do not prevent her from making decisions for herself. She has been married for ten years and has no children. Her husband recently left her, largely because he could no longer tolerate the emotional flatness or unresponsiveness that is caused by her disease; he refuses to give her any money for her support, although he has both a clear legal obligation, and the means, to do so – Mrs N.L.'s husband is, indeed, quite well off financially. Her own family are at present supporting her, but their financial means are limited and they cannot do so indefinitely. She is incapable of working and will soon be forced to seek social assistance. A social worker, who became involved with Mrs N.L. during one of her hospital stays, takes her to a local legal clinic to see a lawyer.

The mental abilities of people who suffer from psychotic diseases often deteriorate when they are placed in stressful situations, and this is true of Mrs N.L. When she first met with a lawyer the combination of her husband's departure and her discomfort over discussing her problems with an unfamiliar person left her so upset that she was barely coherent. The lawyer asked Mrs N.L.'s father to act as a litigation guardian on Mrs N.L.'s behalf, but he has always been afraid of anything to do with the law and lawyers and refused to help. It is clear that Mrs N.L. very much needs a lawyer's assistance, and her claim is a relatively uncomplicated one. Moreover, the lawyer very much wants to help Mrs N.L. but is reluctant to proceed because he doubts her mental capacity to give him valid instructions. He suggests to Mrs N.L. (who accepts his suggestion) that she undergo an assessment of her competency to retain and instruct counsel.

CHAPTER TWO

Incompetency as a human problem

These nine cases illustrate a number of important points that are discussed elsewhere in this book. One extremely important point has already been raised but bears repetition – competency generally becomes an issue in emotionally and spiritually trying circumstances, while people are trying to cope with a host of serious problems that have arisen because they are mentally ill, aging, or have suffered a brain injury. Questions about competency tend to be raised by, and about, individuals who are already angry, confused, or upset by the turn that their life or the life of a relative or friend, has taken. Competency first comes to sight as a difficult, emotionally wearing, *human* problem, and people must therefore address the emotional aspects of incompetency before turning their attention to its more technical medical and legal dimensions. Indeed, it is impossible to comprehend fully the medical and legal responses to incompetency without first grasping the human problems they are meant to address.

Incompetency, especially in people who have a progressive dementia, is often devastating to suffer through or witness. It is an awful thing to watch the progressive deterioration of a relative's or a friend's personality or character, and then to be left with the burden of caring for a being who looks like, but is not, the same person that he or she once was. Everyone has difficulty accepting painful truths, so it is understandable that people often have great difficulty admitting that they are (or a relative or friend is) becoming incompetent and that there is nothing anyone can do to prevent it. People tend to deny the existence of incompetency, or to feel great pain when they do accept its reality. Incompetency is often a great personal loss that arouses the same passions – devotion, guilt, suspicion, and sorrow – that other great personal losses do. People are often emotionally overwhelmed by brain injuries or diseases that deprive them, or someone whom they love, of significant parts of themselves.

The case of Mr P.A., the man whose wife threw him out of the house because she did not realize that his unpredictable behavior was caused by a progressive dementia, well illustrates the emotional pain associated with incompetency. Mr P.A. lashed out verbally at his wife, with whom he had always before had a close and loving relationship, and improvidently spent money on which the security of his family depended. His wife was hurt and angered by his behavior and forced him out of their home. Later, she felt extremely guilty when she learned that his strange behavior was not really his fault. She now also harbors deep grief and anger because her husband is irrevocably slipping away from her, although she is determined to care for him as long, and as best, she can. She is unable to relieve her feelings by talking with him about his disease and their future; he either refuses to talk about such matters or denies that he has any problems. She is uncertain of her own ability to protect her family without Mr P.A., and she is extremely fearful of the future. Mrs P.A.'s complex and contradictory feelings are typical of people who must cope with incompetency. To cope with it successfully, one must understand not only the feelings of the incompetent person but also those of the people concerned with that person's care.

The loss of competency threatens to undo the achievements of a lifetime. What people call maturing, or simply growing up, is a process by which one becomes competent at increasingly difficult, but increasingly satisfying, tasks. It takes years to develop the competencies that permit success in social relationships, at work, in recreational activities like sports, and in solid and rewarding family relationships. Competency is a potent source of self-esteem or happiness. People take pride in themselves, for example, when their work is going well, or when they master a new skill, such as sailing a boat or using a computer. Their pleasure at mastering a new skill is heightened by the recognition and honor that their new competency brings them from others. Anyone who has watched a toddler take a few halting steps, then gaze expectantly up at her parents' beaming faces, will easily grasp this basic truth. Self-esteem depends both on the pleasure people take in their own competency and in the recognition that it brings them from others. When competency begins to fail, not only do people think less of themselves, they also lose their means of attracting recognition and praise from others. It is not surprising that people often react to their own incompetency with intense and painful emotions: incompetency isolates people from themselves and from others.

It can be crushing for a person to learn that he or she is (or is thought to be) incompetent, and for this reason we should be very cautious about challenging another's competency. Questioning competency aims a blow at the person's self-confidence and the security of his or her relations with others. An untrue allegation of incompetency, whether made intentionally or mistakenly, or for good or bad reasons, will certainly cause unnecessary pain and can cause even worse harm. Recall that the issue of a person's competency is often raised by a relative or a friend whom the person trusts. A false accusation of incompetency made by someone close may be viewed by its victim as a betrayal, and it will almost certainly distance the alleged incompetent from his or her accuser. At best, a false accusation of incompetency will produce anger, resentment, or distrustfulness; at worst, it can permanently alienate someone from a family member or a well-meaning friend.

False accusations of incompetence can also have terrible legal consequences. The laws and institutions that are intended to protect people from being wrongly declared incompetent and stripped of important liberties are, in many places, inadequate to the task. Furthermore, even good laws can be misapplied and the people who administer the law are as flawed as everyone else. A false but credible accusation of incompetence can take away part of a person's liberty, for example, if a guardian is appointed to make decisions for a person capable of making them unaided. Such injustice is always deplorable and can have particularly debilitating effects on elderly people. Older people who are capable of living independently, but who are forced against their will to live in, say, a nursing home, often become hopeless. They feel worthless and abandoned and give up doing things for themselves; their abilities atrophy with disuse, and they ultimately *do* become incompetent. A false accusation of incompetency may become a self-fulfilling prophecy.

It is never easy to strike a proper balance between the desire to help incompetent people and the desire to protect competent individuals' liberty and independence against unwarranted interference. It is impossible to do so without having clear ideas about what competency and incompetency are. The goals of respecting liberty and protecting people from harm may often in practice be reconciled by accurately distinguishing competency from incompetency, and by specifying the exact nature and degree of incompetency that an individual suffers from. Those who wish to care well for an incompetent person – and not just professional caregivers like nurses and doctors – must learn how to perform their own, informal, assessments of competency. To do so, however, means distancing oneself from one's own emotional reaction to the signs of incipient incompetency, while maintaining the bond of trust with the ailing friend or relative. Before people can turn to the task of assessment they must first come to terms with their own reactions to others' incompetence. Before undertaking a competency assessment it is first necessary to grasp how incompetency changes the lives of incompetent people and the lives of their relatives and friends.

Dealing with incompetent people

Those who care for incompetent people are often filled with resentment, anger, and fear, and therefore they find it hard to think clearly about what they ought to do or to seek assistance from others. At the same time, they are often overwhelmed by the practical difficulties involved in the care they are giving. Looking after a beloved relative or friend who is, for example, becoming increasingly demented is physically and emotionally exhausting; yet it need not be an overwhelming or unbearable task. Indeed, if people learn what incompetency is; adjust their expectations so that they ask no more than the ailing person is able to give; and take advantage of all the help they can get from their community, relatives, and friends, the burdens of care can be held to a manageable level. In many cases it is even possible to restore and maintain the bonds of friendship and love that are often strained by the onset of the illness. The keys to coping well with a relative's or a friend's incompetency are to first learn what incompetency is, then to become informed about the help available in one's community for people who are incompetent and, finally, to develop a realistic plan for care. With a little knowledge it is possible to cope, and even to cope well, with incompetency.

Shame, fear, and denial

It is very common for people to feel ashamed of themselves when they fail at some task, even though the failure occurred through no fault of their own. For example, people who have lost their jobs often feel ashamed of themselves even if the loss was due to a circumstance, like economic recession, that was completely beyond their control. It is not surprising that incompetent individuals often feel great shame when they realize that they no longer have the abilities (like those required to withdraw money from the bank) that everyone else around them possesses. Mr P.A. is a case in point. Mr P.A. has always been a very independent man, proud of his financial acumen. He came to Canada as a poorly educated immigrant, but with hard work and shrewd investment achieved a fair measure of financial success. Shortly after his wife became aware of his improvident spending she searched his desk and found a large pile of unpaid household bills; Mr P.A. had left these unpaid because he had become incapable of filling out a check. When confronted with the unpaid bills Mr P.A. became angry. His wife inquired whether something was wrong (she thought that he was having an extramarital affair and hoped that he would confess it to her), but he told her to mind her own business. Mr P.A. in fact knew that he was no longer competent to look after the family's finances, and he was certain that something was very wrong with him. However, used to thinking of himself as an independent, capable, and self-reliant man who neither wanted nor accepted help from others, he was unable to accept his predicament or admit to others that he was bewildered and much in need of assistance.

Mercifully, not every case of incompetency begins so dramatically and unhappily. In many cases of dementia or brain injury the person's relatives and friends suspect (even though the person denies having any problem) that he or she is ill and take steps to offer comfort and reassurance. There was little that Mr P.A.'s wife could do to allay Mr P.A.'s fears, because she did not know that he was ill. But Mr P.A.'s feelings are typical of people who are becoming incompetent, and so he probably could have been comforted (as are many people who are becoming incompetent) by a frank but gentle and loving talk with a spouse, relative, or close friend.

How, then, might Mrs P.A., if she had suspected that her husband was becoming incompetent (or anyone else who suspects that this may be true of a friend or relative), help reduce his shame and quiet his fears? Mrs P.A. might have told her husband that he seemed to be unusually upset and then suggested to him that a visit to a physician was the appropriate reaction to his feelings. If he had resisted her suggestion or reacted badly to it (say, by becoming depressed or demoralized), Mrs P.A. could then have explained to him that seeing a doctor was the first step toward locating the cause of difficulties. She might also have made it easier for him to accept help by telling him that she cared for him and would stand by him whatever his problem turned out to be; she might have said further that the help she gave was not burdensome because it expressed her love and gratitude for all he had done for her and their children. Undeniably there are risks associated with revealing to a person – especially a proud and independent one – that someone else is aware of his or her mental difficulties; there are, however, also great risks associated with not doing so, not the least of which is that a remediable problem will go untreated. On balance, people generally should discuss their fears or observations of incompetency in another with the failing person, although they must also exercise good judgment in selecting an appropriate place, time, and manner in which to raise the issue.

Dependency and unreasonable demands

Part of Mr P.A.'s problem is his unwillingness to admit that he needs help. Mr L.H., the man whose children wish him to move to a nursing home, is an example of the opposite emotional extreme. It is true of incompetent people like Mr L.H., as it is true of people generally, that some of them quite readily admit their limitations and accept help. Some people accept help easily because they have always been willing to acknowledge their own needs for, and dependence on, others and have therefore developed strong bonds of trust with those who wish to care for them. Other people, like Mr L.H., accept help easily out of a sense of entitlement to it; people like Mr L.H. are often extremely demanding because they feel that care is *owed* to them. When others fail, as they inevitably do, to meet their heavy demands, people like Mr L.H. become resentful and cease to trust them. Mr L.H. has been very demanding of his daughter from the moment he moved into her home. Now that his daughter is unable to provide for all his needs Mr L.H.'s resentment manifests itself as suspicion and anger; these feelings fuel the accusations of theft and maltreatment that he levels at her and her husband and repeats to others. The problem presented by people like Mr L.H. is to strike a realistic balance between the desire to help them and the caregiver's physical and mental limits.

How is it possible to strike a realistic balance between a faltering individual's demands and one's own capacity for providing care? Those who care for incompetent people sometimes refuse to acknowledge their own limitations, in the same way (and for the same reasons) as incompetent people refuse to acknowledge theirs. The starting point for balancing a caregiver's limitations and another person's needs is to acknowledge the caregiver's limits. Yet often, when people are advised to acknowledge their limits, they react as though they have invited to feign weakness as an excuse for callousness; people sometimes think that acknowledging their limits is the same as abandoning an ill person. The truth is that acknowledging limits, far from being a sign of weakness or callousness, is a proof of strength and good intentions. Those who care for an incompetent person must behave like people who assess their financial means and live within a budget, rather than like people who spend money heedlessly and then suffer for their profligacy; living within one's means – physical, financial, and emotional – is a proof of strength and self-control, a measure of responsibility. People must assess and acknowledge their limits not because they seek excuses to give up caring for ill people, but because they wish to care for them in an intelligent way that they can sustain, if necessary, over a long period.

Not only is it a proof of strength to acknowledge one's limits; it is also strengthening. To restate an important point: a realistic person is not callous or pessimistic. A realistic person assesses things as they are, not as he or she wishes them to be. Indeed, the sooner that people cease reacting to another's incompetency as an object of shame, sorrow, or guilt and treat it instead as something that simply is, the more likely they are to find intelligent and sustainable ways of giving the incompetent person the help that he or she needs. Often, when people move beyond their emotions into a realistic assessment of an incompetent person's predicament, they discover resources of strength in themselves that they did not know they possessed. Realistic people simply refuse to allow their emotions to bully them into arrangements that will, in the long run, fail.

Having arrived at a realistic assessment of his or her own abilities, and of the incompetent person's needs, a caregiver is in a position to take the next step – to learn about and take advantage of the resources that his or her community offers to incompetent people and their caregivers. In Mr L.H.'s case, for example, his relatives considered the possibility of respite care, in which a failing person is periodically admitted for a short hospital visit to give those who look after him or her a short vacation from the burdens of care. A failure to follow this very reasonable approach illustrates the importance of realistically appraising one's limits before reaching them. Mr L.H.'s daughter never questioned her ability to care single-handedly for her father, even when it was apparent to all those around her that she could not continue doing so for much longer. As a result, the possibility of respite care was not raised with Mr L.H. until his dementia was already considerably advanced. Often, as people become increasingly de- mented, already strong traits of their character become even more exaggerated; so it is no surprise that a person like Mr L.H., whose dementia was fairly advanced, and who has always demanded a great deal from his daughter, refused to allow someone else to care for him in her stead for even a short time. Had the possibility of respite care been raised at an earlier stage, Mr L.H. might well have been more receptive to it. Instead, outside help was not sought until the situation had degenerated into a crisis and the available options had become very limited. Good and early planning, always important when caring for incompetent people, is essential when caring for a particularly demanding person.

The emotional toll

The onset of incompetence, particularly in cases of progressive dementia like Alzheimer's disease, can be incredibly hurtful for the family of the demented person. Often a well- and long-loved spouse or relative, who is suffering from dementia, will inexplicably withdraw his or her affection and begin to behave very strangely. This is hard enough to accept when people know that the spouse or relative is ill, but impossible to accept if the emotional withdrawal and other strange behavior seem deliberate. Yet in their early stages progressive demen- tias like Alzheimer's disease can sometimes be difficult to detect. Demented people in the early stages of an illness, like Mr P.A. whose wife threw him out of their house, are sometimes labelled careless or lazy or mean. The onset of incompetence, when it brings inexplicable and hurtful changes in the behavior of a relative or friend, can be crushing. It is important to be honest with oneself when dealing with a person who may be becoming incompetent; people can neither come to terms with another's illness, nor give the ill person any help, until they admit that the ill person is, in fact, ill.

Even people who know that a friend or relative is ill often have difficulty coming to terms with their knowledge. Mrs P.A.'s emotional reactions are typical of people who learn that a spouse or close relative is demented. She cannot accept that her husband is no longer, and will never again be, the man she married and whom she has loved for many years. Previously a loving and attentive husband and father, he is now sometimes unable to recognize her or their children. He frequently wanders from home and becomes lost, so that it is impossible to leave him unsupervised; she resents his increasing dependency, and she is afraid that the ever-increasing expense of caring for him will ruin her financially. She knows that she will not be able to care for him at home much longer, but she feels guilty at the thought of sending him to live elsewhere. Moreover, she is uncertain about where else he can live or even from whom she can seek advice about his care. Mrs P.A. is confused about the practical aspects of life without her husband's advice and help and equally about the nature of her obligation to him. In these feelings she is far from alone. It is impossible to separate the subject of assessment and care from a consideration of the bonds that lead people to undertake the care of vulnerable, weak, and ill.

Why care?

People should strive to provide others with the least-restrictive care possible. Sometimes by doing so caregivers free themselves of the burden of providing unnecessary and unwanted care. In other cases, however, providing the least-restrictive form of care, based on a formal or informal competency assessment, may sometimes impose extra demands on the caregivers. Most important though, in practice, care of any description, let alone well thought out and respectful care, is often available only to incompetent people whose relatives and friends are willing to provide it or to help obtain it. The provision of care – and especially of the least-restrictive alternative form of care – often involves personal sacrifices by relatives and friends.

Why should people compromise their own happiness and independence only to make incompetent people happier and more independent? Why should people, for example, provide the least-restrictive form of care if it is easier not to do so? What is the nature of the obligation that people have to their weak and failing relatives and friends; why is it just for the strong and healthy not only to care, but to care respectfully, for the weak and ill? The indisputable fact is that many people feel a powerful obligation to care for their incompetent relatives and friends, and they derive considerable satisfaction from discharging this duty well. The question of obligation is best approached by returning to the starting point of this book: the human needs of incompetent people and of those who care for them.

There are many reasons why people wish to be cared for by their relatives and friends rather than by professional caregivers and why people provide respectful and loving care to those close to them who have become incompetent. Two principal and related reasons stand out. First, many incompetent people think that their relatives and friends will see them as whole human beings, and fear that professional caregivers will not or will not be able to do so. Second, the administration and reception of care is a way (not always successful) or bringing a proper finality to friendships and loves and thus harmony and meaning to our lives.

Care by family and friends

People do not want to be thought of as merely a case, a technical problem to be solved by a specialist who views them in the narrow perspective of a discipline. For example, people commonly fear that if it is necessary to choose between their death and the imposition of extreme or heroic medical treatment, the decision will be made by someone basing it strictly on medical criteria, rather than on a combination of medical criteria and knowledge of the patient's character and desires. This fear is not entirely groundless, for what seems to a specialist the right thing to do may not be the right thing for a particular individual. Many people want decisions to be made for them by someone who views them as a whole; people's illnesses or incompetence, even if overwhelming, are not all there is to them. Incapacity does not cancel out entire lives; in some important matters the best decision cannot be made for people simply by applying technical standards. It is an exercise of humanity to make important decisions for oneself, and if this is impossible, to have them made by a relative or close friend.

To many people it seems that allowing professional caregivers to make decisions for an incompetent person is simultaneously a betrayal of the incompetent person and a self-betrayal. The explanation for this feeling lies in a powerful combination of memory and gratitude. In the presence of an elderly or incompetent relative or friend, people often reminisce about the past – with the person if he or she is capable of it, and by a kind of internal dialogue with their own memories if he or she is not. Memories in turn may remind them that they are caring for a human being to whom they owe gratitude. This is particularly true of the relation between elderly parents and their children. When people care for their elderly parents they acknowledge them as the source of their own lives; in a sense people see in their elderly parents the same humanity that their parents saw in them as children when they were young and helpless. Human beings do not cease to be worthy only because they have lost their full human powers. If people allow their relatives and friends to be treated in an impersonal or uncaring way they acknowledge the meaninglessness of their own past with the person, and indeed the meaninglessness of their own futures: what right has a person to expect decent and respectful treatment themselves if they do not provide it to others? When people care for an individual who is unable to care for himself they honor the person, their own memories, and their hopes for their own futures.

Conversely, if people deny, in theory or in practice, the existence of an obligation to treat the weak and helpless as human beings, they threaten their own humanity. Those who treat the weak callously imply that their obligations to one another depend entirely on mutual usefulness and that incompetent people (or, more precisely and frighteningly, those who are deemed by some authority to be incompetent) are of no human consequence. When people care for the old and weak they assert the dignity of human life; when they discard or ignore the old and weak they threaten that dignity. Underlying the desire to care for the elderly and incompetent is the moral intuition that life itself is good and that it remains so even when a person is incapable of exercising all of his or her human faculties.

Gratitude and finality

People want their lives and relationships to end satisfactorily; this means, in part, that they want to feel that their intimate relationships were more than just random happenings, the significance of which dies with them. They want a shape to their lives, and often find it by acknowledging and rewarding those who have been important forces in their lives. Unfortunately, people often fail to grasp the extent of their debts until after their benefactors are dead. Many of us experience, at least once in our lives, the peculiar mixture of gratitude and regret, completeness and dissatisfaction, that arises on acknowledging, too late, the help that we received from another. The gratitude and completeness arise because we feel that there is alive in us some aspect or element of the dead person, who would be pleased by what we have become; regret and dissatisfaction arise when we have failed to express our gratitude to our benefactors while they were alive. The desire to acknowledge those who have shaped our being, and to be gratified in turn by their recognition, is sometimes felt powerfully and appropriately among friends but is more commonly felt among relatives – especially between parents and children.

When caring for incompetent individuals, people receive in return an opportunity to acknowledge and repay their debts to the living, which is preferable to paying those debts later in the form of memory and regret. In short, those who care for the incompetent are often motivated by gratitude – by the desire to help those who have helped them – and so to bring the relationships to a satisfying conclusion. There seems to be, for example, a natural order or harmony in the progress of the generations that has children care for their parents, only to be cared for in turn by their own children. But why does this bond among the generations seem so natural? When people care for those who have cared for them they establish a tradition, a moral link among the generations, and thereby achieve a kind of immortality. When the weak, especially elderly or dying parents, are cared for by the young and strong they know that a being who is fundamentally like themselves will remain alive and active in the world after they are gone. Those who provide care prove that they have mastered their parents' lessons, and they may hope that just as some part of their parents remains alive in them, some part of them will similarly remain alive in their own children. The provision of care to the weak is a natural activity because it provides satisfaction to both recipient and giver; the weak are recognized as human beings worthy of honor and respect, and the strong display their gratitude and often have the pleasure of its acknowledgment. But most important, both the weak and the strong secure a sense of the meaning and continuity of their own lives. There is great satisfaction in providing proper care to incompetent relatives and friends.

Independence and contradictions

The desire to provide respectful care for incompetent people is not only deeply rooted, but it also forces people to recognize and foster their independence; the desire to provide care is based on reciprocal gratitude between the weak and the strong, and such a relationship can exist only among independent and self-willed human beings. People cannot force others to be grateful to them, but only to feign gratitude. Implicit in the desire to care is the recognition of independence. Competency assessment, and the care based on it, are elaborations of the natural impulses that cause people to want to care for others. But although there are powerful natural impulses that make people want to do the right thing, there are also powerful impulses that work in the opposite direction. When people understand that they are the objects of conflicting principles and desires, they are truly in a position to grasp the importance of well thought out plans of care for incompetent people.

Because they value life, because they value tradition, and because they value those who have helped to shape their lives, people feel obliged to care for individuals who are incompetent. Care is a valuable activity because it brings a kind of happiness, but people also desire other kinds of happiness. On the one hand it is inhuman to ignore the needs of incompetent relatives and friends; on the other hand, if people were to devote themselves solely to their incompetent friends' and relatives' care they might not have and raise their own children and so would interrupt the very tradition that requires them to care for the elderly. The same humanity that calls people to the aid of those who are incompetent also requires them to realize their own capacities and abilities in independent activity, including caring for their young. When caring for an incompetent person or planning for their own care in the event of their incompetency, people must balance an incompetent person's need for care with their own needs.

Giving and receiving

It is often difficult in practice to strike a balance between a caregiver's needs and those of an incompetent person. Those who struggle to cope with other responsibilities (such as family and job) while providing for the needs of an incompetent person will at some point almost certainly become frustrated or exhausted and lose sight of their higher principles and deeper feelings; everyone is prone to confusion. Indeed, the tendency toward confusion is natural both because there is a real conflict between the needs of caregivers and individuals who are incompetent, and because feelings toward relatives and friends are often clouded or ambiguous from the outset.

In all human relationships, but particularly in family relationships, there is simultaneously give and take; human beings try to satisfy one another's needs. But even in healthy families, whose members respect and care for one another, there is often tension; it is rare for people to be completely satisfied with their children, siblings, or parents. Often this dissatisfaction clouds judgment when dealing with a relative who has become incompetent; sometimes it makes people unwilling to give, or, conversely, sometimes it deprives people of the ability to know when they have given enough. Moreover, feelings of dissatisfaction with family and friends are almost always exaggerated by illness or incompetency; this is particularly true of the relationship between parents and children. As people near the end of their lives they attempt a summing up, an emotional finality in their relationships; yet human reality often resists this desire for completeness, and people often discover that a complete resolution is impossible – for example, sometimes it is impossible to overcome or forget a lifetime of disagreements. As well, deaths and illnesses are very much individual experiences, and dying or incompetent people commonly feel profoundly alone and become quite withdrawn. Some individuals who are near death or incompetency become resentful of those who are not. It is hardly surprising that people often feel a haunting sense of incompleteness on the death or incompetence of a parent, relative, or close friend. At the same time as being called on to make sacrifices for a friend or relative, they must often come to terms with their own unfulfillable needs and desires.

When the multitude of conflicting principles, needs, and emotions that make up one's attitude toward the incompetent is recognized, it becomes easier to grasp the importance of planning for care. To achieve the goal of appropriate care, it is essential to remove as many obstacles to it as possible. Prudent people will plan, while their minds are relatively clear and they are relatively disinterested, to lessen the burden of providing care; they will plan for their own incompetence. Failing this, the next best approach is to formulate, at the earliest possible moment, a plan of care for a person too incompetent to make his or her own. All human beings are likely to become incompetent at some point in their lives; self-aware people must come to a sober acceptance of their weaknesses and needs, whether in requiring care or in experiencing difficulty in delivering it to another. It is an expression of sobriety, maturity, and intelligence for a person to make a reasonable plan for his or her own incompetency or for that of another.

Basic concepts

Task-specific competency, task-specific care

Sometimes people do become completely, or almost completely, incompetent and require total or very extensive care that involves the appointment of a guardian. But in many cases incompetency is only partial. The general rule is that the care provided to a partially incompetent person should correspond to the nature and extent of his or her disabilities and needs and thus minimize the loss of his or her right to make independent decisions. Incompetency is often task-specific, and so too are its remedies.

This book describes two different kinds of competency assessments: informal and formal. An informal assessment, which may be conducted by a non-professional (even by a relative or friend of a person who may be incompetent), is intended to determine only whether there is sufficient justification to seek a full-blown competency assessment from a professional assessor. Informal assessment may be thought of as a preliminary investigation. Its purpose is to identify an appropriate response to a perhaps incompetent person's needs, but not to determine whether a person is, in fact, incompetent. In contrast, a formal competency assessment is conducted by a professional assessor, such as a psychologist or psychiatrist; it often has significant legal ramifications; and it should determine authoritatively whether a person is incompetent. These two kinds of assessment are described in greater detail below, and a separate chapter is devoted to each. At this point it is sufficient to understand that there is more than one kind of assessment; either may reveal that a person requires a certain kind of help to perform a particular task, and so may provide an exact prescription for that person's care. Even when an assessment does not result in a prescription for care it is often an indispensable step toward formulating one. For example, if a formal competency assessment reveals that the problem underlying a person's financial incompetence is an impaired memory, those who care for the person will then know that they should seek appropriate memory aids for that person. The beginning of proper care is a proper competency assessment.

The least-restrictive alternative

The care of incompetent people, like their assessment, begins with the concept of task-specific competency and incompetency. In theory this means that people should always seek to provide an incompetent person with the form of care that both adequately meets his or her needs and restricts his or her liberty as little as possible. This may seem like a daunting command to apply, but in practice there are many relatively simple means of satisfying it. The least-restrictive alternative for an incompetent person's care may often be discovered simply by paying attention to the person's own wishes and by exercising some common sense. For example, a person may while competent have expressed formally (as in a general durable or enduring power of attorney) or informally (as in a conversation with a son or daughter) some desires about the kind of care that he or she wishes to receive in the event of incompetency. In such a case, the least-restrictive kind of care will be that which the incompetent person himself or herself requested while competent to do so.

Unfortunately, many people become incompetent without having expressed their own wishes regarding their care. In other cases, people have expressed wishes that are unrealistic or that a caregiver is unable or unwilling to meet. In such cases people may receive important clues about the least-restrictive form of care by considering the incompetent person's reactions; often the least-restrictive alternative form of care is also the one that makes an incompetent person happiest and most vigorous. For example, a person who has become incompetent to manage his own finances might still be competent to execute an enduring power of attorney and might have firm views about who should manage his finances for him.

Mr F.C., who did not trust his wife to manage his finances, is such a person. His chosen attorney is his grandson, who is an accountant. Knowing that his grandfather is financially incompetent, this grandson must now decide what form of care is appropriate for him:

1   He can allow an official from the local adult protective agency to assume control of his grandfather's finances.

2   He can follow his grandfather's wishes (as expressed in a legally valid general durable power of attorney) and himself assume control of his grandfather's finances.

3   He can apply to have a court declare his grandfather incompetent and to appoint him (the grandson) or someone else his grandfather's financial guardian.

In some states and provinces there are two distinct forms of guardianship – financial and personal. Thus, even if Mr F.C. is deprived of the right to make financial decisions he will retain the right to make decisions about his personal care. In some places a financial guardian is called a 'conservator,' acknowledging the limited obligation to manage the person's finances and conserve his or her property. In some jurisdictions a form of guardianship called 'limited guardianship' is also available; in these jurisdictions the law allows or requires the judge who appoints a guardian to tailor the guardian's power to accommodate the functional disabilities of an incompetent person (often called a ward). Under a limited guardianship law, for example, a guardian may be given the power to make medical decisions for a person but not the power to decide where she will live.

Armed with all this information the grandson considers how best to follow the principle of the 'least-restrictive alternative.' He knows that some intervention in his grandfather's life is unavoidable. He also knows that his grandfather will hate losing control of his finances to a public official when a trusted member of his family could instead manage them. As well, the grandson has a close and strong relationship with his grandfather, and will, unlike a public official, be able to make decisions that approximate those his grandfather would make if competent. When it is impossible to make decisions on the basis of a 'substituted judgment' the grandson knows he is more likely than a public official to make decisions that will please his grandfather. Finally, the grandson will be willing to consult more frequently with his grandfather than a public official likely will be, and he has training and experience that equip him to manage his grandfather's finances effectively. Public trusteeship is clearly not the least-restrictive alternative for Mr F.C. This conclusion leaves the grandson a choice between acting as his grandfather's attorney pursuant to his power of attorney, or becoming his guardian. Guardianship may be necessary in the long run – if, for example, the grandson must eventually make medical decisions for Mr F.C. or choose his place of residence. At present, however, Mr F.C. requires only financial assistance. A guardianship application would humiliate Mr F.C.; on the other hand, a court order would give the grandson unassailable authority, and it is possible that someone might later challenge Mr F.C.'s capacity to execute a power of attorney. However, the psychiatrist who assessed Mr F.C. is quite convinced that he has the capacity to execute a power of attorney and has prepared a detailed report of her reasons for thinking so. By thinking about his grandfather's own wishes and needs, and applying his common sense, the grandson concludes that the least-restrictive means of providing for the management of his grandfather's finances is for him to assume control of his grandfather's finances under the authority of an enduring power of attorney.

Good planning is essential

There are cases where it is difficult for practical reasons to identify and adopt the least-restrictive alternative form of care. Such difficulties are often unnecessarily compounded because people have unduly delayed, or avoided, the process of planning. Incompetent individuals and their caregivers too often find themselves facing a predicament simply because nothing has been done until the deterioration is very advanced or some crisis has erupted. In such cases, caregivers often find they must resort to very restrictive, or otherwise ill-considered, forms of care. In other cases caregivers fail to take their own needs and limits into account; they take on too much, exhaust themselves, and ultimately engage in a frantic search for any form of care that offers them a desperately needed respite. People who wait too long to make a realistic plan for their own care, or for the care of a relative or friend who is becoming increasingly incompetent, are likely to have fewer – and less desirable – options available when they do begin to plan.

To sum up, undue delay in planning care often results in unnecessary loss of liberty and independence. Early planning is a key to the least-restrictive possible care, and the best early plans are generally those made by people for themselves while they are competent to do so. This kind of planning is best done with a full understanding of competency assessment, and it is dealt with in chapter 7 of this book.

CHAPTER THREE

Assessing competency

Three truths constitute the foundation for thorough, fair, and accurate competency assessments.

1 Incompetency (also called incapacity) means the absence of the capacity to make choices or decisions.

2 Competency is not a single ability that people either have or lack. People use different abilities to make different kinds of choices, and so they may be competent to make some decisions but incompetent to make others. Competency is task-specific.

3 Competency assessments must look at the whole individual. The fact that a person has a mental illness, a mental handicap, or a brain injury, or has performed poorly on standard psychological tests, generally does not prove that he or she is incompetent. A person is incompetent only if mental deficiencies make it impossible for him or her to make a decision or decisions that he or she must now (or must soon) make. In practice, incompetency arises only when a person is no longer able to function in the circumstances of his or her own life.

Simply put, competency has to do with abilities to make choices or decisions and must be assessed in relation to the particular decisions that particular individuals are actually called on to make.

Ability to make a choice

A competent person is capable of choice. But what is a choice? Mr P.A., (the man who is suffering from a rare form of dementia), for example, squandered his money and spoke abusively to his wife. In some sense he wanted to do what he was doing. But did he *choose* to behave as he did? At one point his wife believed that he had. She thought that he no longer loved her and suspected him of infidelity. When Mrs P.A. learned that her husband's behavior was caused by a disease she no longer thought that he had deliberately hurt her. Mr P.A.'s illness has deprived him of the ability to control his behavior. Even now, when his dementia is very advanced, if he is asked whether he should spend all his money or spend some and save some, he answers that the latter choice is better; yet if he is given any money, he immediately squanders it. Mr P.A. acts on impulse rather than thought; he is incapable of making choices about what to do with his money and about many other things as well.

When people *choose* to do something, their thoughts and their actions go together. Imagine, for example, that Mr P.A. had no progressive dementia but was deliberately squandering money that his family needed for its support on an extramarital love affair. Many people would describe his actions as wrong, or bad, or callous, thereby implying that Mr P.A.'s behavior was deliberate; he would be seen as having the ability to behave well but not doing so. However, a person who knows that Mr P.A. suffers from dementia would likely use a morally neutral term (like incompetent) to describe Mr P.A.'s actions, thereby implying that his behavior was not deliberate; he would be seen as unable to behave any differently than he does, unless someone prevents him from acting on his impulses. Mr P.A. is incompetent because his actions are beyond his control. Although incompetence is a judgmental and hurtful word, unlike the words wrong, bad, and callous, it says nothing about a person's moral character. It describes only the ability to harmonize thought and action – to make *choices*.

Task-specific competency

A competency assessment inquires into whether a person is capable of making his or her own choices. But how may choice be distinguished from impulse? The answer to this question has many parts, and it will emerge slowly throughout this book. The starting point is to think about the kind of choices that people commonly make and the abilities they need to make them. For example, a person who can neither add nor subtract would be an incompetent bookkeeper. But if this incompetent bookkeeper has very quick reflexes and good eyesight, he might very well be a competent racing car driver. Similarly, Mr P.A.'s neurologist, who knows that competency is task-specific, is certain that Mr P.A. is financially incompetent but does not therefore assume that he is incompetent to execute a power of attorney. Indeed, Mr P.A.'s neurologist knows that different abilities are needed to decide who will manage one's finances than are needed to actually manage them oneself. Incompetency may be partial: a person who is financially incompetent may still be capable of selecting a substitute financial decision maker. Although there is good reason to question Mr P.A's competence to execute a power of attorney, the neurologist is unwilling to conclude that he is incompetent to do so. Instead, she decides only that she has ample justification to refer Mr P.A. to a psychiatrist for an assessment of his competence to execute a power of attorney. A proper competency assessment focuses on the specific abilities that an individual needs to make decisions in the specific circumstances of his or her own life.

Assessing the whole individual

To do that, a proper competency assessment must provide an accurate picture of an *individual's* capabilities and deficiencies. An assessment may involve medical assessment and diagnosis, but the mere fact that a person has an illness, handicap, or disease does not prove that he or she is incompetent. Nor is it proper to conclude that a person has lost some ability only because people with the same medical problem generally do. A competency assessment that focuses on the individual's diagnosis, rather than on the individual's abilities, is not really an assessment but an exercise in statistics.

In most cases a diagnosis of mental illness, mental handicap, or brain injury, or a poor performance on a standard psychological test, is insufficient reason to conclude that a person is incompetent to perform a specific task. The same illness, handicap, or injury may affect different people in markedly different ways. The consequences of events that may impair or damage the brain vary with the nature of the event, the person's character, the kind of life that person has led, and the kinds of assistance (whether from professional service providers or relatives and friends) available. For example, to be competent to execute a power of attorney a person must understand the nature of the document. Many people with the same disease Mr P.A. has would be incompetent to execute a power of attorney because (among other things) the disease often impairs the ability to learn, thus making it impossible to inform a person properly of the meaning and significance of the document. But Mr P.A. once had his wife execute a power of attorney giving him the power to sell, while she was away on vacation, some property that they jointly owned. Mr P.A. thus has a general understanding of a power of attorney, based on his earlier experience with one, and so *may* be competent to execute one. With his prior experience Mr P.A. may be competent to execute a power of attorney, even though many other people suffering from an inability to learn would be incompetent to do so.

A person should not be labelled as incompetent to perform a particular task without an assessment of his or her particular strengths and weaknesses. Knowing that someone has a mental illness, a mental handicap, or brain damage is often a good reason to be concerned about that person's competence, but it is seldom sufficient reason to conclude that the person *is* incompetent.

Competency assessments thus must focus on abilities rather than diagnoses; they must focus also on the reasons that people give for their actions. A person is not incompetent only because he or she does things that many people find disagreeable or difficult to understand. Indeed, it is very easy to confuse strongly marked traits of character with incompetence. Often acts that would be taken as a mark of eccentricity or independence in a young and vigorous person are wrongly taken as proof of incompetency in someone who is old or ill. A competency assessment must therefore ask what kind of person is being assessed and what sorts of things the person has generally held to be important. An incompetent person is so not merely because he or she fails to behave as others wish him or her to, but because he or she cannot behave in accordance with his or her *own* considered or habitual standards of behavior.

The case of Mrs R.H. (the woman who was hospitalized with a broken hip and whose physician does not want her to return to her own apartment) shows how important it is to pay careful attention to the reasons that people give for their actions. Mrs R.H.'s physician, for example, thought that no rational person would willingly expose herself to the risks that Mrs R.H. wanted to run. But Mrs R.H. is, and always has been, a very independent and private woman who hates to be watched, let alone supervised, by others. She has lived alone for a long time and has always preferred solitary and reflective activities, like reading or listening to music, over social ones. The thought of any form of group living, particularly in a supervised environment, is abhorrent to her; Mrs R.H. would, quite literally, rather die than surrender her privacy and independence. Given the kind of woman that she is it is hardly surprising that Mrs R.H. prefers a risky but independent life to a safer but less independent one. Mrs R.H.'s decision may or may not be a good choice but it is a valid one that she has the right to make for herself. An individualized competency assessment must consider the whole person and not just his or her present behavior; what matters in competency assessment is whether a person's choices make sense judged according to that person's own considered or habitual standards or goals.

Caution in challenging competence

There are at least five good reasons for being cautious about challenging another's competency.

1   Competency assessment often involves a searching investigation of a person's abilities and thoughts. Many people dislike opening intimate aspects of themselves and their lives to inspection by strangers; competency assessment can be humiliating or upsetting.

2   Even when people welcome a competency assessment (as they sometimes do) it is still an invasion of their privacy.

3   Merely raising the issue of someone's competency can be hurtful or damaging to them.

4   Eccentricity and incompetency are easily confused, and it is easy to wrongly challenge the competency of someone who is merely eccentric.

5   The desire to help someone who appears to be at risk of harming himself or herself makes it easy to wrongly assess the person as incompetent.

There are many reasons why a person may wrongly be found incompetent. It is important to remain constantly aware of how easily an assessment may go astray and to consistently follow strategies that encourage thorough, careful, and fair assessments. Principal among these strategies is the division of competency assessment into a two-stage process. The first stage is called informal assessment and the second is called formal assessment. In practice many of the same procedures and issues arise in both kinds of assessment, but the goals of the two kinds are different. Before elaborating on the difference, it is necessary to reconsider the human context in which incompetency generally becomes an issue.

Competency tends to become an issue when other people fear that someone is incapable of conducting some aspect of his or her personal affairs without somehow harming himself or herself or others. When people challenge another's competency they usually do so because they want to intervene somehow in that person's life, even if the person does not want them to. Often the motive for a competency assessment is to determine whether a person should be deprived of his or her ordinary rights. Given the many ways that an assessment can go wrong, and the harm frequently done merely by challenging another's competency, it is important not to do so without very good reason. Regrettably, those who challenge another's competency often think that the onus is on the person to prove that he or she is in fact competent. This book rests on the view that the onus is on those who allege that another is incompetent – first, to show that there is good reason even to investigate that person's competency, and then to prove that the person is incompetent if this is in fact the case. Informal assessment is the process by which people ask themselves whether there is sufficient reason to investigate another's competency. Informal assessment also sets the stage for a formal assessment of competency by pinpointing those areas or tasks in respect of which a person is likely to be incapable. Informal assessment is intended to prevent people from wrongly challenging others' competency; it is also intended to limit the scope of any ensuing formal competency assessment.

In an informal assessment, the people involved do not examine so much the person whom they think may be incompetent as their own knowledge of that person and his or her recent behavior. An informal assessment should always precede a formal one, except in cases of manifest incompetency (as when a person is in the final stages of Alzheimer's disease). For example, a hospital physician may be told by a patient's nurse that the patient is incompetent to decide where she will live. That is not enough reason to subject the patient to a formal assessment of her competency to choose her own residence. Instead, the physician should ask the nurse to explain the reasons for her concern, and she should ask herself whether there is good reason to think that the patient may well be incompetent.

Similarly, consider a child who is caring for an elderly parent who refuses to move from her own home to a nursing home. The child thinks that such a move is in the mother's best interest, and she is considering seeking guardianship of her mother and moving her to the nursing home against her wishes. Before seeking a competency assessment leading to her mother's guardianship, the daughter should ask herself whether an objective person would agree that there is reason to think that her mother is incompetent to decide where she will live. Both the daughter and the physician in the other example given above should ask themselves whether the issue is a simple dis-agreement about what is in a person's best interest (in which case no formal competency assessment is required) or whether the person really may be unable to make his or her own choice (in which case a more formal assessment is justified). Informal assessments do not necessarily involve the use of tests or invasive examinations (although in a medical or personal care institution they may involve both), and they may be conducted by anyone.

In practice many of the same issues arise in both formal and infor-mal competency assessments, but there is one significant difference between the two. With informal assessment people simply ask whether a fairly searching investigation of another's competency is in order; the outcome of this decision will likely have no immediate implication for the other person's liberty. Formal assessment, in contrast, is conducted only by trained assessors, often but not always psychiatrists, and may have immediate implications for the liberty of a person who is found to be incompetent. By seeking a formal assessment people indicate that they are prepared to deprive the assessed person of the opportun-ity to make some or all of his or her own decisions.

There is one other distinction between the formal and informal assessment of a person's competence. In informal assessment people weigh their own views, often without revealing them to anyone else and certainly without revealing them to the person who may be incom-petent. In contrast formal assessment involves, in three related ways, going public with one's doubts about another's competency.

1   Having decided that there is reason to investigate another's competence it is necessary to seek the assistance of a professional assessor and to share with that assessor the reasons for thinking that the person is incompetent.

2   To seek the assistance of a professional assessor of competency is to invite him or her to intervene in the allegedly incompetent person's life.

3   Most significantly, in seeking a formal assessment of competency it is necessary to reveal one's doubts about a person's competency to that very person.

The decision to seek a formal competency assessment, regardless of the outcome, may humiliate or upset the allegedly incompetent person. A formal assessment of competency can have a dire effect on a person's life, and so should be performed only if it is really necessary. Excepting only cases of manifest incompetency and emergencies, an informal assessment of competency should always be carried out before a formal one is requested.

Medical treatment and assessment

It is of crucial importance not to confuse formal competency assessment with ordinary medical care. A formal competency assessment occurs when a person is examined by a professional assessor specifically to determine whether he or she is capable of making decisions. Medical care, in contrast, is the evaluation of a person's physical status to determine whether that person is suffering from an illness or disease, especially a treatable one. It is a serious matter, to be approached cautiously, to conclude that a person's behavior is evidence of incompetence; on the other hand, it is simple prudence to encourage a person whose behavior is sufficiently worrisome to seek medical attention. For example, the appearance of confusion and disorientation in a person does not necessarily mean that a competency assessment is called for, but it is certainly a good reason for suggesting a check-up. Indeed, the check-up may actually become part of an informal assessment of competency, for it may eliminate the possibility that a person's unusual, worrying, or disturbing behavior has a medically treatable cause. If a person displays behavior or symptoms that would ordinarily lead a prudent onlooker to suggest that the person seek medical care, it is perfectly reasonable to suggest, even if that person is fully competent, that he or she see a physician.

Admittedly the distinction between medical care and competency assessment sometimes breaks down in practice. This is especially so when a person imprudently refuses to seek medical care. In many circumstances such a refusal is a sufficient reason for seeking a formal competency assessment, for example when a person is known to suffer from an illness that may affect competency. Even when there is no evidence of incompetency, a refusal to see a doctor may be a sufficient reason to approach a physician for advice. Doing so may, of course, lead to a formal competency assessment. For example, the physician may encourage a relative or friend of the confused person to take legal steps to compel the person to accept an unwanted medical assessment. When there is conflict between the desire to avoid an unwarranted intrusion into a person's life on the ground of incompetency and the need for medical care, it is generally wise to resolve the dilemma in favor of medical care. The reason is that medical care may reveal that the abnormal behavior is caused by a treatable condition. The rule of avoiding unwarranted challenges to another's competency should not be applied so dogmatically that it becomes a barrier to the provision of essential medical care.

CHAPTER FOUR

Informal competency assessment

Informal assessments determine whether there is good reason to think that another person may be incompetent. Such assessments can be, and are, performed by many different people in many different circumstances. Later in this chapter some detailed cases of informal assessment will be presented, but it may be helpful at the outset to offer examples of common situations in which informal competency assessments are often performed.

- Lawyers who prepared wills for elderly people often attempt to satisfy themselves that their clients know what a will is, want to make one, and are a capable of coming to decisions about the distribution of their property.

- Physicians, nurses, and other health-care professionals who provide in-home services to elderly patients whose capacity for thought and action are clearly impaired must often determine whether their patients remain capable of caring for themselves.

- The relatives and friends of stroke victims must often decide whether the stroke has deprived them of the abilities needed to continue living alone or to continue managing their own finances.

- Physicians who care for people whose mental abilities are clearly impaired and who refuse life-sustaining medical treatment must decide whether the refusal is a legally valid one that must be followed.

In short, informal competency assessments may be performed by a wide variety of people and in a wide variety of settings. There are, however, three elements common to these examples, and, indeed, to many other situations that call for an informal competency assessment.

1   The assessor comes to the assessment with some background knowledge of the person who is to be assessed and of a decision or decisions that the person is actually being called on to make.

2   On the basis of his or her knowledge of the person the assessor has good reason to *raise the issue* of the person's competence, but insufficient proof to conclude that a formal assessment of competency is called for.

3   The assessor has good reason to think that, if indeed incompetent, the person may be at risk of harming himself or herself, or others.

Often it is a relative or friend who raises the issue of another's competence. This is hardly surprising, since those who are closest to a person will have the best opportunity to recognize changes, perhaps when they are still subtle, that suggest the presence of mental deterioration or disability. It is entirely appropriate for family members to raise the issue of a relative's competency (or for a close friend to raise the issue in the absence of family) and entirely possible for them to do so in a careful and responsible way. But it is also possible for such allegations to be wrongly made, with unfortunate consequences both for the person who makes it and for its subject. Indeed, this simple truth applies not merely to relatives and friends, but to anyone who challenges another's mental competency. Informal assessment is a process – a way of thinking about competency – that recognizes the dangers of challenging another's competency and that encourages people to clarify and examine their reasons for doing so before they take any step (say, a psychiatric assessment of competency that may lead to a guardianship application) that may have drastic consequences for another person's well-being.

Questions to ask

Informal assessments usually involve the following questions.

1 What is the problem? The first step in informal assessment is to state clearly the problem that has made an assessment necessary. Often by clarifying the problem people become aware of solutions to it that do not require a competency assessment. If, for example, Mrs R.H.'s physician had clarified the specific risks that Mrs R.H. was subject to he might have thought of reasonable alternatives to a formal competency assessment and involuntary residence in a nursing home. The risk of a fall while showering, for example, could be alleviated by installing a wall bar and hand shower that would permit Mrs R.H. to shower while seated, and to get into and out of the tub safely. The risk of a kitchen fire could be alleviated by the purchase and use of a microwave oven. Perhaps Mrs R.H. would even give up cooking if a hot meal were delivered to her every day by a meals-on-wheels program. Similar measures could be taken to eliminate the risk that Mrs R.H. would set a fire while ironing her clothing – she could, for example, have her clothing pressed by a cleaner or purchase permanently pressed clothing. Perhaps Mrs R.H. would simply agree to wear wrinkled clothing if this allowed her to remain safely in her own apartment. There is often more than one way to address the problems of an incompetent or failing person, and a competency assessment should begin by questioning its own necessity.

Moreover, until people have clarified the problem that they wish to address (and the kind of care that others appear to need) they cannot know what kind of assessment must be performed. Competency is task-specific. There is, for example, no reason to assess a person's capacity to make health-care decisions when only competence to select a place of residence is at issue. To get the right kind of assessment people must first clarify the areas in which a person is at risk.

2 Will a competency assessment help solve the problem? Before concluding that there is no alternative to a formal competency assessment, people should decide what kind of assistance they think is needed and satisfy themselves that it can be provided. Too often competency is challenged unnecessarily, only to discover (perhaps even after the person has been declared incompetent) that the kind of help that is needed is unavailable. For example, a person who is living in dangerous circumstances may be found incapable of choosing her own place of residence only to discover that no alternative residence is available for her. Merely finding someone incompetent is no guarantee that he or she will receive help; competency assessment is useless unless accompanied by a solid plan for assistance.

3 Is a voluntary solution practical? Even if a person manifestly requires some kind of assistance, that does not mean a competency assessment is justified. It is first essential to determine whether someone who obviously requires a particular kind of care (for example, help with bathing) will accept it voluntarily. There are many reasons to prefer voluntary over forced arrangements for the care of incompetent or failing people. The first, and strongest, is that voluntary arrangements are often the best way to reconcile the sometimes inconsistent goals of preserving well-being while respecting a person's right to make his or her own decisions; the provision of care that a person both wants and needs protects well-being *by following the person's own decisions.* Second, informal, voluntary arrangements are often more successful than involuntary ones which the person who is being helped resents and tries to undermine. Finally, informal arrangements are often much less expensive and emotionally wearing to establish than formal ones; it is, for example, extremely unpleasant (and sometimes expensive) to go to court 'against' a relative or friend to seek a guardianship order, even if the action is well intended and justifiable.

As a rule of thumb, care that can be provided without a formal assessment of competency is preferable to care that cannot be. But like most rules of thumb, this one must be applied flexibly and with due attention to individual circumstances, not like a moral principle that must be strictly obeyed. There are, for example, people who are so impaired that a formal incompetency assessment leading to guardianship is manifestly the only way of providing adequate care for them. Another caution: it is important to avoid imposing care, without the lawful authority to do so, on a person who is merely too passive or timid to resist it, or on an incompetent person who is incapable of consenting to it. This caution applies with special force to medical treatment or personal care that cannot be administered without informed consent, either of the person who receives it or of someone authorized by law to consent for an incompetent person. There are nonetheless many intermediate degrees of willingness to receive assistance between resolute and implacable refusal of help and passive willingness to accept it, and much room for originality in providing it.

4 What is the law? The kind of care that people may provide to an incompetent person will often be determined by the local laws. To determine whether it is sensible to challenge another's competency it is important to learn (certainly before seeking a formal competency assessment) something about the law of incompetency in the relevant state, province, district, or territory. This will almost always require the advice of a lawyer or of a health-care professional who has experience in dealing with incompetent people. Although a comprehensive survey of the legal mechanisms by which decisions may be made on behalf of incompetent people is far beyond the scope of this book, it is possible to discuss some of the most common legal devices (such as durable powers of attorney and guardianship) that are available in many North American jurisdictions.

It is particularly important to learn something about the available legal mechanisms for substitute decision making before assessing a person whose ability to manage some aspect of his or her life (often finances) is clearly impaired or diminishing. The principle of the least-restrictive alternative applies to assessments; it requires that they be tailored to enhance independence and allow people to make their own decisions where possible. Imagine, for example, that an informal assessment confirms that a person is having difficulty managing his or her finances. An assessor whose legal knowledge is limited might assume that the logical next step is a formal competency assessment leading to the appointment of a financial guardian. An assessor who has some legal knowledge might, however, consider whether the person is capable of executing a general durable power of attorney. Instead of concluding that a guardian should be appointed, such an informed assessor will consider maximizing the person's independence by inviting him or her to consider the possibility of voluntarily selecting and empowering a substitute decision maker. If the person *chose* to follow this course of action, the assessor could then refer the person to a lawyer and conduct (or have an appropriate professional conduct) an assessment of the person's competency to execute a power of attorney. In such a case the judicious use of informal assessment will allow the subsequent formal assessment to serve the positive and libertarian purpose of allowing the person to choose his or her own substitute decision maker, as opposed to the negative and restrictive imposition of a substitute on a recalcitrant subject.

The law of substitute decision making can be divided into two general parts.

1   Legal devices, such as the durable power of attorney, allow a competent person to decide who will make decisions for him or her

if he or she becomes incompetent. These may be called 'voluntary' legal devices.

2   Legal devices, such as court-ordered guardianship, allow a person to make decisions on behalf of an incompetent person who may not have sought (and who may even reject) his or her assistance. These may be called 'involuntary' legal devices.

A common voluntary legal device is the enduring or durable power of attorney. A common involuntary legal device is the judicially ordered guardianship of the person or property of a mentally incompetent person. There is a place for both voluntary and involuntary legal devices in the care of incompetent people and even in the care of the same person at different times. For example, people like Mr P.A. (the man who squandered his money) who have a progressive dementia often know early in their disease that they are incompetent. Such people may want help but are too ashamed to say so. If a general durable or enduring power of attorney, that is, one that applies to the management of property and not to medical or other personal decisions, is suggested to someone like Mr P.A. early in the dementia and as an exercise of choice rather than an admission of weakness, he or she will often welcome the opportunity to execute one. It is important to inform people like Mr P.A. that they, and they alone, have the power to decide who will become their attorney and what powers the attorney will, and will not, exercise. As well, people who execute a power of attorney should be told that they generally retain the right to make their own decisions, and even to revoke the power, so long as they are mentally competent to do so. Once incompetent, however, the person can neither make his or her own choices nor revoke the power; but even in this case the principal will have the comfort of knowing that he or she, and no one else, decided who was going to make substitute decisions.

At some times, and for some people, it is simply not realistic to consider a voluntary legal arrangement like the execution of a durable power of attorney. There are, for example, stages to the progress of dementia. In some stages dementia may reduce inhibitions and cause people to behave aggressively. When Mr P.A. squandered a great deal of his money his dementia had progressed to the point of depriving him of his ordinary inhibitions. At that time he would certainly not have voluntarily given his wife, or anyone else, the power to make financial decisions for him, although if approached at an earlier time he might have done so. During this aggressive stage of his illness it might have been justifiable to appoint a financial guardian to manage Mr P.A.'s affairs; in a still later stage of his disease such an aggressive approach might not be necessary because Mr P.A., if approached in a frank but gentle way, might then agree to execute a durable power of attorney, assuming of course that he was competent to execute one. Like most other decisions that people must make about their dealings with others who are (or who may be) incompetent, the selection of an appropriate legal approach calls for the exercise of judgment rather than the application of iron-clad rules.

5 Whose interest is being served? A formal competency assessment should be sought only if it serves the incompetent person's interests. There are three generally accepted standards for determining whether a competency assessment will serve someone's interests. The first, and best, standard is direct or indirect indication from the allegedly incompetent person of the circumstances in which his or her competency should be challenged. A mother, for example, might tell her daughter that if she becomes too ill to manage her own home she wants to be moved to a nursing home; if the daughter later has doubts about her mother's competence to live independently she will know that an assessment of her mother's competence is in her mother's interests according to her mother's own competent wishes. The second, and less desirable standard, is that of substituted judgment. Applying this standard involves putting oneself into the mind of the allegedly incompetent person and asking what that person would decide if competent to do so. Thus a son who is trying to decide whether he should assess his father's competency with an eye to becoming his guardian and moving him to a nursing home might consider that his father has always considered it a matter of great importance to impose no burden on his children and that caring for the father at home is becoming very burdensome indeed. But in many circumstances people do not know what an allegedly incompetent person's wishes were previously, and are unable to approximate them. In these cases people must apply the third, and least satisfactory, standard for determining best interests: they must ask themselves what a reasonable person in the allegedly incompetent person's position would want to have done.

When applying the 'reasonableness' standard of best interests it is important to guard against the all-too-human error of assuming that what is in our own best interests is therefore also in the other person's best interests. Recall here that competency assessments often take place in an emotionally charged atmosphere. People who challenge another's competency are often so confused and upset that they are incapable of self-examination. To make a hard matter harder, in competency cases, as in many other emotionally messy human affairs, it can be extremely difficult for even a scrupulous and emotionally detached observer to know whose interests are served by a particular course of action. The case of Mr L.H., whose children wish to place him in a nursing home, is one such morally ambiguous situation. It is reasonable to argue (as a competent Mr L.H. probably would) that his children are simply serving their own interests by seeking a formal competency assessment to justify a guardianship order and his place-ment in a nursing home. But it is also reasonable to argue (as Mr L.H.'s son-in-law probably would) that a formal assessment of competency will serve his own, his wife's, *and* Mr L.H.'s interest alike; if Mr L.H.'s daughter becomes (as is likely) totally incapable of caring for Mr L.H., he will then be much worse off than he will be if he moves into a nurs-ing home now, while she is still able and willing to help care for him.

In competency cases the search for the pure motive is often fruitless and paralyzing. If people find that they cannot analyze their own motives, or if they know that their motives are mixed, they should shift from self-analysis to analysis of the needs of the person whom they wish to assess; they should also focus on defining and considering reasonable alternatives to a competency assessment. In some cases an informal assessment itself may be the best way to resolve the dilemma of murky or conflicting interests. It is vitally important to articulate conflicting motives or considerations and to remain alive throughout an assessment to the possibility that judgment has been colored by self-interest.

6 What risks are involved in the present situation? One major purpose of an informal competency assessment is to decide whether there is sufficient evidence to justify a formal assessment. This process involves asking two questions.

1   Is there objective reason to think that a person is at risk of harm-ing himself or herself or others?

2   If there is objective evidence of risk is the risk confined to the

person himself or herself, and does he or she *choose* to run it – aware of the foreseeable consequences of the decision to do so?

To answer the first question it is necessary to examine the person's life, to specify the kind of harm to which he or she is exposed, and to assess the likelihood that harm will actually materialize and its likely gravity if it does. Differently put, the task is to judge what is likely to happen to a person if he or she continues to live as he or she now does. The second question asks whether a person has the ability to appreciate and accept risk, that is, is the person capable of *choosing* to run a risk.

Assessing risk

How much risk is too much?

The phrase 'at risk' simply means that there is a chance of suffering an injury or loss. The world is full of risks to life and limb; driving an automobile on the highway, riding a bicycle, and playing sports are all risky activities, yet no reasonable person would say that someone is incompetent because he or she is a traveling salesman, a bicycle courier, or a professional football player. Risky conduct, as such, is not proof of incompetence. The initial problem in competency assessment is to distinguish tolerable risks, ones that are insufficient to justify a competency assessment, from intolerable risks, ones that do justify the performance of one. Risk assessment is an art, not a science, because it involves the exercise of judgment, but that does not mean that it is a subjective or arbitrary exercise. A mere feeling or intuition that a person is at risk is at best a starting point for risk assessment, and it is not a valid ground for challenging the person's competency. A competency assessment is called for only if some of the objective hallmarks of intolerable risk are present in a given individual's life. Absolutely certain risk assessments are beyond human reach, but precise and justifiable ones are not.

As with informal competency assessment in general, the assessment of risk involves a series of questions.

1 Is the risk new or old? The first question to ask in an objective assessment of risk is why it is necessary to perform such an assessment *now*. What recent changes in a person's life have aroused concern about his or her well-being? If there have been no such recent changes, if the person has (for example) merely continued to do something risky that he or she has done for a long time without suffering serious harm, that suggests that there is insufficient risk to justify an assessment of competency. For example, Mrs R.H. (the woman who was hospitalized with a broken hip) is said to lack the abilities to bathe, iron, and cook and so to be at risk of harm. But she has lived alone for many years without injuring herself while bathing or setting a fire while cooking or ironing. The fall that brought her into hospital had nothing to do with bathing, ironing, or cooking; rather, she slipped on ice while walking outside – an accident that has, at some time, befallen almost everyone who lives in a northern climate. It is generally fair to treat past performance as indicative of future performance, barring some good reason for holding otherwise. Unless something has recently changed in Mrs R.H.'s life, such as deterioration of her mental condition or eyesight, that has adversely affected her abilities to bathe, iron, and cook, her physician does not have sufficient reason to conclude that she is exposed to intolerable risk if she continues to live alone. Mrs R.H.'s physician has made a very common error; he has given his own speculative judgment more weight than he gave to objective evidence of Mrs R.H.'s ability to live on her own without serious mishap.

2 Are there concrete instances of failure? The best evidence of abnormal risk is manifest instances of failure that are distressing to the failing person. For example, Mr P.A., the man whose wife forced him out of their home, has always run the household financial affairs and prides himself on his financial acumen. When his wife found a desk drawer full of unpaid bills and learned that he was inexplicably squandering large sums of money, she had compelling evidence of abnormal financial risk. There are three reasons why evidence of this kind is compelling. First, because it shows that something new and bad is going on in Mr P.A.'s life; his behavior is unprecedented and has caused real financial harm to him and to his family. Second, because it is manifest evidence of risk; unlike Mrs R.H., who has never suffered the harm that her physician says she is risking, Mr P.A. has now actually failed to conduct his finances properly. Most important, Mr P.A.'s conduct is a failure according to his own habitual standard of judgment; he has always prided himself on his financial self-sufficiency, and there is no reason to think that he has changed his mind about the value of financial prudence. Given the kind of man that Mr P.A. has always been, it is difficult to imagine him voluntarily running a grave risk of financial harm. Just as past success may fairly be taken as indicative of future success, past failure may fairly be taken as indicative of future failure.

3 How grave is the risk? A person is not at abnormal risk if he or she fails at just any task; rather, the failure must expose the person to harm that will make his or her life significantly worse than it now is. In other words, the graver the anticipated risk, the more likely it is to be intolerable. For example, if Mr P.A. was able to write checks in payment of his household bills, but sometimes forgot to date them, that would hardly qualify as a risk of financial harm, let alone as an intolerable one; the worst imaginable consequence of an undated check is that it will be returned and that some interest will have to be paid on a bill that was outstanding until a proper check was submitted. Risks that are of little significance are hardly intolerable and are not proper grounds for challenging someone's competency.

4 Is the risk imminent or remote? Even when a person is prone to some kind of failure, and the consequences of a failure will likely be grave, he or she may still be capable of taking steps to reduce risk to tolerable levels. For example, in the case of Mr N.C. (the young man who was injured in a motorcycle accident) a bad financial decision could deprive him of any hope for a relatively happy and independent life. But Mr N.C. recognizes this risk and so will accept assistance in the management of his finances; he is prepared to rely on any financial adviser whom his parents select, and he also wants his parents to help him with day-to-day financial matters like the payment of his bills. So Mr N.C. may not actually run an intolerable financial risk if he becomes more involved with his own financial affairs, because he recognizes the risks to which his increased involvement will expose him and is willing to protect himself against them. A risk will generally not be intolerable if it is unlikely to materialize in the actual circumstances of a person's life.

5 What is the risk of harm to others? A classic formulation of individual liberty is that it ends when one person's action threatens to harm others; the right to swing your arm ends at the tip of the next person's nose. Competent adults are allowed to run risks for themselves, but they are not allowed to impose them on others. A risk that someone could freely choose to impose on himself on herself may be intolerable if imposed on others. Mrs R.H.'s physician, for example, might acknowledge that the actual evidence of Mrs R.H.'s incompetency is relatively flimsy, but could still plausibly argue that a thorough investigation of her competency is in order because if she sets a fire it will place every inhabitant of her apartment building in jeopardy. Or, what would be a very minor financial failure (like forgetting to date checks) in a person who looks after his or her own affairs, might constitute an intolerable risk for someone who works as a bookkeeper and is responsible for the proper handling of other people's money. Risk must be assessed with regard both to the individual, and to others whom he or she might harm.

6 How objective is the assessment? It is sometimes extremely difficult to assess reliably the risks faced by someone (like a parent, sibling, or good friend) whom the assessor loves and feels responsible to protect. The problem is that the acceptance of responsibility for another's safety sometimes causes people to apply a much too conservative standard of acceptable risk. Judgment may be clouded by the powerful combination of the natural desire to protect weak or vulnerable people with the equally natural desire to avoid any personal blame or guilt should these people actually come to harm. Bluntly put, sometimes there is confusion between the desire to avoid guilt or blame and any objective evidence of risk. This does not mean that people are forbidden to assess the risks faced by someone they love; in many instances relatives and friends are best situated to know when someone is at risk of harm, simply because they have the opportunity to observe the person regularly in the circumstances of his or her daily life. But there is an obligation to be especially skeptical of any conclusions made that a close friend or relative is at risk of harm.

In practice, a good way to discharge this obligation to be skeptical is to seek the opinion of a third party who has no special emotional investment in the matter. This third party need not be a health-care professional, but can be any reasonably sensible and disinterested person. Before seeking this outside opinion the assessor should formulate his or her reasons for believing that a friend or relative faces an intolerable risk of harm; it is often helpful actually to write the reasons out, for the very act of recording a view often brings a measure of objectivity. In any event, the more clearly that the reasons are formulated, the easier it will be for an outsider to assess them. Another reasonable approach to the problem is to discuss the matter with a psychiatrist, or some other health-care professional, who has experience at assessing competency and to seek his or her opinion about the desirability of a formal competency assessment.

7 Is a risk chosen or accidental? If a person is indeed running an intolerable risk of harm that alone may not make him or her incompetent. *Incompetency is the inability to make choices. A competent person chooses to run risks; an incompetent person simply happens to run them.* A very important factor in risk assessment is whether the person has voluntarily, and with awareness of the potentially adverse consequences, chosen to engage in a risky activity. Competent people do sometimes continue with an activity that has caused them harm in the past, and may well do so again in the future. For example, during the 1988 summer Olympics the American diver Greg Louganis struck and lacerated his head while executing a dive, yet he continued diving (very successfully) in the competition. Louganis's actions displayed courage, not mental incompetence; he voluntarily risked injury in the pursuit of something that he valued more highly than his safety – an Olympic victory. Mrs R.H., the woman who wishes to live independently but whose doctor believes that she is incapable of doing so, is also a brave person; she is prepared to run risks for the sake of something that she values more highly than her safety – her privacy and independence. So, if Mrs R.H. is prepared to give up any behavior that might pose a risk to others – that is, if she will stop using stove burners or an iron – she is neither at intolerable risk herself nor is she imposing such risks on others. People can normally decide for themselves whether they wish to accept or avoid a risk; a risk to oneself alone that is voluntarily assumed, with recognition of the potential consequences, is not an intolerable risk. The goal of risk assessment is *not* to place others in a cocoon, but only to make certain that their choices are their own and that they cause no harm to others.

Summary

Intolerable risk comprises six distinct elements.

1   A change in the person that impairs his or her ability to protect himself or herself, or others, from harm.

2   Evidence of manifest failure.

3   The gravity of the anticipated harm.

4   The imminence of the anticipated harm.

5   The imposition of risk on others.

6   The inability to choose to run a risk.

Risk assessment involves striking a balance among these six discrete elements. In some cases all six elements may be present, in others only one or two. For example, a risk that is not particularly grave might be intolerable because it is very likely to occur. Or a risk that is not very likely to take place might be intolerable because it is extremely grave. Although there is an art to risk assessment, it is not an arbitrary or capricious exercise. There is a solid and rational structure to risk assessment that involves identifying and quantifying the objective evidence of the presence of risk.

Competency assessment in general, and informal assessment in particular, require the exercise of judgment. There is no such thing as a perfect competency assessment, but there are good and bad ones. A good informal competency assessment is task-specific, necessary, likely to lead to the person's receiving help if he or she is found to be incompetent, properly respectful of the individual's own choices, and focussed on the objective risks that the person faces. These requirements may, in the abstract, seem complicated, but they are little more than a recipe for the exercise of common sense. To prove the point consider, as exercises in informal assessment, three of the cases that were introduced in chapter 1.

Three informal assessments

Mr L.H.: A formal assessment is required

Mr L.H.'s children want to become his guardian so that they can choose his place of residence. They have sought a reasonable alternative to guardianship but have failed, for Mr L.H. will accept neither a move to a nursing home nor respite care. Other family members are unwilling, or unable, to help care for him. The only local day-care program for the elderly will not accept people like Mr L.H., who are incapable of attending to their own bodily needs. Public in-home nursing assistance is available only to people who live alone or whose relatives are physically unable to care for them. The only alternative to home care of Mr L.H. by his daughter is institutional care in a nursing home, and the only way to place Mr L.H. in a nursing home is to become his guardian. His children have spoken with a lawyer, and they are aware of and prepared to meet a guardian's legal obligations. They have visited several nursing homes and have found one that is well run and that expects to have a bed available soon; there is thus an alternative residence available to Mr L.H. if he is found to be incompetent. The children know that Mr L.H. will be enraged when he learns of their intentions. However, the situation in their home is so intolerable, and Mr L.H. is already so extremely distrustful, that a competency assessment followed by a guardianship application cannot make things much worse than they already are.

When the children meet with their lawyer he asks them to give him concrete reasons for thinking that Mr L.H. needs a guardian. They answer that he cannot attend to his own basic bodily needs. He is incapable of making appropriate use of the toilet or of devices to control his incontinence. He is clearly unable to feed and clean himself properly, or even keep track of his personal possessions without assistance. Moreover, he could not possibly cope with a medical emergency or a fire, as he is incapable of locating and dialling telephone numbers. Mr L.H.'s well-being depends on his daughter's assistance, yet his behavior makes it very difficult, if not impossible, for his daughter to give him the help that he needs. It appears that he understands neither his own dependency nor the effect of his behavior on others. It is also clear that he does not choose to behave as he does. Mr L.H. has always been a very demanding, but also a very loving, father; it is very out of character for him to accuse his daughter of theft, let alone to do so publicly. Mr L.H. cannot understand that his behavior threatens his daughter's health and makes it impossible for him to continue to live in her home; it is therefore extremely unlikely that his behavior will alter for the better. There is good reason to believe that Mr L.H. cannot decide where it is appropriate for him to live, and so to refer him for a psychiatric assessment of his competency to choose his place of residence.

Mrs R.H.: No reason for a formal assessment

Mrs R.H. was hospitalized when she broke her hip after slipping on some ice outside her apartment building. She wishes to return to her apartment. Her physician, however, feels that she will be unsafe at home and strongly believes that it is in her best interest to move to a nursing home. Although he is prepared to challenge her competence formally he prefers not to do so. He meets with Mrs R.H., hoping to convince her to enter a nursing home voluntarily.

The physician points out to Mrs R.H. that she has already fallen once and broken her hip; that she was confused and disoriented while in the hospital; that she almost fell while showering; and that she left an iron burning and misused the stove during her assessment by the occupational therapist. She replies that she has lived alone for many years without harming herself and believes that people are making a great deal of fuss over events that mean very little. The fall that brought her to hospital was a freak; she walked outside early one morning, without realizing that the temperature had dropped below freezing the night before, and slipped on a small patch of ice. Had she walked out one hour later the ice would probably have been melted. During the early part of her hospital stay she was, she admits, confused and disoriented; she attributes her impaired mental state to the painkiller she was taking and to being in unfamiliar surroundings. At home, in her apartment and familiar neighborhood, she is never disoriented. She also admits that she did almost fall in the shower, but says that this was before she had fully recovered from the effects of her fall. Her physical stability has been greatly improved by therapy, and she is now able to shower without difficulty. As for the problems with appliances, she challenges the validity of the OT's conclusions. She (Mrs R.H.) never uses an iron anyhow, and cooks only with a toaster oven, precisely because she knows that her hands are unsteady, and she fears that she might accidently start a fire. It is often difficult to tell when someone is making excuses to cover up a disability, either from embarrassment or from a desire to keep others from interfering in his or her life. Mrs R.H.'s claims, however, are plausible and supported by objective evidence (her fall took place in late fall before winter was firmly established; she was given a powerful painkiller that is particularly likely to confuse an elderly person; her walking has improved considerably; she at present shows no signs of disorientation or confusion). The physician is impressed by the intensity of her desire to return home. It is clearly painful for her to reveal intimate details of her life to him, yet she is willing to do so because she wants to convince him that she should return home. She evidently hates institutional life, and a nursing home would be a misery to her. The physician concludes that Mrs R.H. is capable of recognizing and accepting any risk of harm to which her solitary life exposes her.

The doctor rethinks his concerns in the light of what Mrs R.H. has told him and concludes that the only valid reason for challenging her competency is the fear that she will set a fire and thereby harm others. He presses Mrs R.H. on this point, and she repeats that she has no iron, and never uses her stove. He asks her whether she would allow a social worker to telephone her landlord and have him disconnect her stove; she says that this is unnecessary, but agrees to the proposal. She agrees to have an OT visit her apartment and make recommendations to improve its safety; all agree that the principal purpose of this home visit is to eliminate any potential sources of fire. She also agrees to accept a monthly visit from a social worker. The doctor concludes that there is no reason to proceed with a formal assessment of her competency.

Mr N.C.: An alternative to competency assessment

Mr N.C. is the young man who became a paraplegic after a motorcycle accident. His parents are his legal guardians, and Mr N.C. feels that they interfere too much in his life. Mr N.C.'s psychiatrist arranges to have a social worker interview the parents. The social worker reports that the parents are well meaning and loving people, who are deathly afraid that if their son regains control of his finances he will impoverish himself and ruin his chance of living a relatively happy and independent life. Moreover, the parents' fears are reasonable. Mr N.C. will have a very large sum of money, and he has never before had to make financial decisions of the kind, or gravity, involved in the ongoing management of a large sum. His brain injury makes it hard for him to master new skills, and some skills that he will require if he is to manage his own money (such as performing basic arithmetic and keeping careful written records) have been impaired by his accident. It is also true, however, that no one really knows exactly what Mr N.C. is capable of doing because he has had no opportunity to live independently since his accident. Mr N.C., the psychiatrist discovers, readily acknowledges his difficulties and is willing to accept help. However, he dislikes the stigma associated with guardianship, and he feels that having a legal guardian would tell the whole world that he is inferior to other people. His principal desire is to choose the location of his new house and to have a small amount of money to spend at his own discretion. He also wants to make financial decisions on the advice of an investment counsellor.

The psychiatrist thinks that Mr N.C.'s parents do not recognize that he has recovered to the point were he can make independent decisions, but also that Mr N.C. wants to take on more than he can handle. For example, even if he receives investment advice he is incapable of assessing its quality, and he would find it very hard to make certain that his instructions are followed. The psychiatrist invites parents and son to meet with him and discuss the situation. At the meeting Mr N.C. tells his parents that he wishes to choose the location of his own house and to have a reasonable amount of pocket money. He says that he will take advice from a financial adviser on investments, and he wants his parents' help with day-to-day matters like the payment of bills. The parents, after some discussion, agree that Mr N.C. can choose the location of his own home and that he should have a monthly allowance to spend as he pleases. They balk, however, at giving him immediate control of his settlement money; they argue that he is clearly not yet ready to handle the money and will, in any event, have to give them some measure of legal control over his funds so that they can help him with day-to-day financial management. They counter his proposal with the suggestion that they establish a trust to hold the settlement money. (A trust is a legal arrangement in which one person holds money, or other valuable things, on another's behalf.) With some help from his parents and the psychiatrist Mr N.C. is able to comprehend what a trust is, and he even makes some suggestions about terms that should be incorporated in the trust agreement. For example, he wants to receive a copy of the bookkeepers's monthly report on the status of his trust funds. His father also offers to have a monthly meeting with his son during which he will explain to him what is being done with his money. On these terms Mr N.C. consents to the establishment of a trust. If matters go smoothly for six months the parents and Mr N.C. will bring a joint application to terminate the guardianship order. It is agreed that the father's lawyer will set up the trust and that Mr N.C. will have an independent lawyer to advise him. The psychiatrist tells the family that he can see no need for a further assessment of Mr N.C.'s financial competency.

An outline of informal competency assessment

This outline is addressed to all those who find themselves undertaking an informal assessment of competency. Often people who undertake such an assessment find it relatively easy to grasp the basic principles of assessment but hard to decide when they have sufficient reason to seek a formal one. To help people who are struggling with this question, a number of these rules identify situations in which a formal competency assessment either should or should not be sought.

General rules

1   *Always* seek medical care for a person who is, or may be, becoming incompetent notwithstanding the risk that this may precipitate a formal assessment of competency. The primary goal of competency assessment is to respect and preserve individual liberty; it in no way preserves individual liberty to leave a person suffering from a treatable illness that is making him or her incompetent.

2   Before undertaking an informal assessment it is important to ask whether it is truly necessary. An assessment is unnecessary if there are adequate alternative solutions to a person's problems.

3   An informal assessment of competency should be performed only if it will serve the interests of the assessed person. It should not be performed if it will serve only the interests of other people. If it is unclear (as it often is) whose interests the assessment will serve, it should be performed only if there are objective grounds for thinking that the person is at risk of harm unless someone intervenes in his or her life.

Situations where formal assessment is always justifiable

1   A person should always be formally assessed if he or she wants to be, so long as the person understands that the assessment might conclude with a finding of incompetency.

2   A person should always be taken for a formal assessment of incompetency if it is an unavoidable precondition for doing something that he or she wants to do – such as executing a power of attorney or making a will – so long as he or she understands that the assessment might conclude with a finding of incompetency.

3   A person who has already been found to be legally incompetent (for example, someone for whom a court has appointed a guardian or whom a physician has certified as financially incompetent) should always be taken for a formal assessment if he or she wishes to challenge the finding of incompetency.

When to avoid a formal assessment of competency

1   A person whose behavior has always been eccentric or unusual, and simply continues to be so, is not incompetent. Eccentricity is not incompetency, and mere disagreement with the way that a person chooses to live his or her life is no reason for a competency assessment.

2   People must guard against the natural desire to save someone whom they love from harm (and themselves from guilt or blame) by exaggerating the degree of risk to which the person is exposed and so justifying unnecessary intervention in the person's life. An assessor whose desire to protect a person may have colored his or her assessment of risk should ask an impartial person to review his or her conclusion that the person is at risk of harm and should be subjected to a formal assessment.

3   A formal assessment of competency should be performed only if

a finding of incompetency will likely make it easier to obtain necessary care for the incompetent person. For this reason it is often helpful to seek the advice of a lawyer, or of a health-care professional who is familiar with the needs and problems of incompetent people, before seeking a formal assessment.

4   A formal assessment should not be performed if the harm to which a person's behavior exposes him or her is slight, or very unlikely to occur, or if the person has *chosen* to run a risk that does not expose others to harm.

When to seek a formal assessment of competency

1   As a general rule, it is appropriate to seek a competency assessment for people who are at significant risk of harming themselves or others, *and* who refuse to accept voluntarily the help they require to avoid causing harm, *but only if* a formal finding of incompetency will make it easier to prevent the person from exposing himself or herself, or others, to harm.

2   It is appropriate to seek a formal competency assessment for a person who has been diagnosed with mental illness, mental handicap, or brain injury, and who is behaving in a quixotic or out-of-character way that exposes him or her to harm.

3   It is appropriate to seek a formal competency assessment for a person whose behavior has already caused harm to himself or herself or to another, and who is unable to recognize the problem or to accept the kind of help required to avoid repeating the harmful behavior.

4   It is appropriate to seek a formal competency assessment for someone who is at serious risk of harm, and who appears to be unable to recognize that this is the case or who is incapable of taking steps to remedy the situation.

5   It is appropriate to seek a formal competency assessment for someone who continually engages in behavior that threatens the well-being of others, and who refuses or is unable to acknowledge that

his or her behavior poses a threat to others, or to accept the help that he or she requires to remedy the problem.

6   Any of the following factors may alone be sufficient to suggest that a person is exposed to an intolerable degree of risk:

a The person's exposure to risk has increased because of recent changes in his or her life.

b The person has actually suffered harm.

c The person would ordinarily avoid risky behavior that he or she now engages in as, for example, when a frugal person suddenly becomes a profligate spender.

d The person's behavior exposes others to a risk of harm, and he or she is unwilling or unable to modify it.

CHAPTER FIVE

Formal competency assessment

This chapter is about the formal assessment of competence. Unfortunately, there are as yet no widely accepted standards for formal competency assessment and practice varies widely. Different groups of health-care professionals have different ideas about what an assessment should involve, and even members of the same professional group may perform competency assessments differently. Readers should not be surprised to find that they, or their friends or relatives, receive a competency assessment that is quite different from those described in this chapter. This chapter serves two purposes: First, to describe the kind of psychological testing that is a common and valuable part of competency assessment, but the worth of which is often considerably overestimated. Second, and more important, to describe the methods and procedures for assessment that have been developed in the Competency Clinic at the Baycrest Centre for Geriatric Care. The Competency Clinic's approach to assessment has been proved both fair and useful. In summary, this chapter is a guide to what people might reasonably expect to find, or to demand, in a formal assessment of a relative, friend – or themselves. It is also offered as a guide to those who perform assessments.

Basic concepts

The previous chapter dealt with the informal assessment of competency. An informal assessment is usually (but not always) conducted privately by a concerned relative or friend, or by a health-care professional, who is not certain whether or not to make his or her doubts regarding a patient's competency known to the patient and whether or not to seek further specialized competency assessment. Informal assessment focuses on the assessor's knowledge of the patient and the patient's life, and it is usually conducted without the aid of useful (but often invasive) medical and psychiatric tests and procedures. Informal competency assessment usually has no immediate legal consequences, although its results may lead to a formal competency assessment that does. In contrast, a formal assessment of competency is conducted by a health-care professional or professionals, is often much more intrusive than is an informal assessment, and may be used as evidence to justify depriving the assessed individual of the right to make his or her own decisions. In Ontario, for example, the physician who performs a formal assessment of a psychiatric patient's financial competency has the power to issue a certificate that places control of the patient's financial affairs in the hands of an official called the public trustee. More commonly, the physician or other health-care professional who performs a competency assessment does not have the authority to override immediately the assessed person's rights, but does provide a report that later justifies another person's doing so. For example, psychiatrists often provide assessment reports on which a judge relies when deciding whether or not a guardian should be appointed to oversee the assessed person's affairs.

To summarize, there are three principal differences between informal and formal assessment. Informal assessments are often performed by people who have no training in assessing competence, but formal assessments are conducted by health-care professionals. Informal assessments are generally not particularly searching or invasive, but formal assessments may involve a wide variety of medical, psychological, and functional tests. Finally, informal assessments usually do not have immediate legal consequences, but formal assessments often do.

There are also some crucial similarities between informal and formal competency assessment. A formal competency assessment, like an informal one, should be necessary, task-specific, likely to lead to the person's receiving help if he or she is found to be incompetent, properly respectful of the individual's own choices, and focused on the objective risks that the person faces. The major advantages that formal assessors bring to competency assessment are a broad base of professional training and experience, access to a range of sophisticated diagnostic tools, and a better knowledge of community resources available for the care or assistance of partially incompetent people than others are likely to have. Well-trained professional assessors, such as psychiatrists and other physicians with relevant training and experience (among them geriatricians who specialize in treating elderly people) and clinical psychologists can go deeper into the causes of incompetency than laymen can, and they have better knowledge of its remedies.

Who performs formal assessments?

There are, speaking very generally, two distinct aspects to a thorough and fair formal assessment of competency: the medical-psychiatric and the functional. Although thorough and fair assessments incorporate both aspects, many assessors now offer only one kind of assessment or the other, and different aspects of the assessment are often conducted by different kinds of health-care professionals. An introduction to the two kinds of assessment is also therefore a good introduction to the different kinds of assessors. The medical-psychiatric aspect of an assessment seeks to determine whether a person is suffering from some impairment of his or her mental processes, and, if so, the exact nature and extent of the difficulty (for example, a loss of memory) and its cause (for example, a vitamin deficiency). In contrast, functional assessment, which is the core of a proper competency assessment, seeks to determine how well a person actually performs various tasks in the circumstances of his or her own life (for example, whether a person is able to do his or her own banking). Medical-psychiatric testing will often reveal that a person has a particular weakness or deficiency, and may give cause to investigate a person's competency, but in most cases only a functional assessment can conclusively determine that a person is incompetent.

As a general rule medical tests are administered by or under the supervision of physicians. Psychological tests that identify and quantify problems of thought and understanding are commonly administered and interpreted by psychologists and psychiatrists, although they are also sometimes administered by occupational and speech therapists and by social workers (depending on local laws and on the practices of different institutions). A broad range of professionals is involved in performing functional assessments, including physicians, psychologists, nurses, social workers, occupational therapists, and speech therapists. A thorough and fair formal assessment of competency often requires a high degree of interprofessional cooperation. An example of an assessment involving such cooperation is included in this chapter.

Legal and medical competency

In some areas, such as wills and guardianship, the law has its own definitions of mental incompetency. In the past, legal definitions of incompetency have tended to be vague or ambiguous, and many still are. For example, a typical Canadian guardianship law defines a 'mentally incompetent person' as someone 'who is suffering from such a disorder of the mind, that he requires care, supervision and control for his protection and the protection of his property.' A comparable American definition defines an incompetent person as someone who suffers from a mental illness, or a disorder, etc. to 'the extent that he lacks sufficient understanding to make or communicate responsible decisions concerning his person or management of his affairs.' These indisputably vague definitions do not give the judges who apply them much guidance in distinguishing incompetency from other problems (such as poverty or ignorance or sheer stubbornness) that can also leave a person in need of protection. Even though more recent legislation incorporates definitions that are much clearer than these two examples, a definition cannot alone convey a complete picture of what competency is or how it should be assessed. Moreover, in many competency cases, and even in those decided under laws that embody clear and justifiable definitions of competency, judges and lawyers rely heavily on medical or psychiatric evidence; in practice, legal incompetency often is what competency assessors say that it is.

If competency assessments accurately distinguish those who need help from those who do not, any ensuing legal proceedings will likely do so as well. But if competency assessments are inaccurate it is extremely likely that any ensuing legal proceedings will also be. Accurate competency assessments protect individual liberty, but inaccurate ones threaten it; accurate competency assessments protect individuals who need help, but inaccurate ones may deprive them of it. Professional competency assessors thus have a significant power over their patients' lives. If individuals' rights are to be protected against unwarranted interference, and incompetent people are to be protected from the consequences of their disabilities, not only must legal proceedings – such as guardianship applications – be conducted thoroughly and fairly; so too must the competency assessments that often determine the outcomes of the proceedings. Those who perform formal assessments of competency bear an onerous duty to protect their patients' liberty and well-being.

The formal assessment process

First steps

Once it is determined that someone's competence should be formally assessed, that person must then be persuaded to accept the assessment. Unfortunately people often arrive at an assessor's office without having been told why they are there. But secrecy of this kind is almost always wrong, often very hurtful to the person who is kept in the dark, and usually futile. Health-care professionals are generally subject to a legal obligation to seek the consent of their patients to a competency assessment, and so they must tell the person what they intend to do before they do it. Someone who is not told in advance about a competency assessment will first learn of it from a total stranger. This is a recipe for producing confusion and distrust in the person who is to be assessed, and it surely makes it much more difficult, if not impossible, for assessors to perform their work thoroughly and fairly. Most important, it may alienate the patient from his or her relatives; it will almost certainly undercut the trust that sometimes makes it possible to devise consensual arrangements that will adequately protect a partially incompetent person. Distrust may lead to an otherwise avoidable guardianship application or some other forced intervention in the patient's life.

People commonly give three reasons for failing to inform someone that he or she is to be assessed.

1   They do not know what to say to the person who is to be assessed.

2   They fear that the person who is to be assessed will become confused or upset.

3   They fear that the person will refuse to cooperate with an assessment if given an opportunity to do so.

A person who needs a formal competency assessment should generally be told so as gently and respectfully as possible. The goal is to convince the person that an assessment is in his or her best interests. For example, one might say to a friend, 'I would like you to go for a competency assessment because I am worried about you. You sometimes seem to be confused or upset about things, and I would like to know why – I am sure that you want to also. I want to help you, but I cannot unless I know what kind of help you need.' As for the fear of confusion, people are more likely to become confused if told by a stranger that their competency is to be assessed than they are if told the same thing by someone familiar whom they trust. Finally, the fear that a person will refuse to be assessed is generally exaggerated; if given a frank, gentle, and respectful explanation of why they should accept a competency assessment, most people do accept it. But even if a person is likely to refuse an assessment little is gained by keeping it a secret till the last minute. Someone who is going to refuse an assessment will likely do so regardless of who suggests it, and will ultimately simply refuse to cooperate with the assessor.

It is indisputably true that some people (including those who manifestly are incapable of caring for themselves) do sometimes refuse a competency assessment. Often this occurs because others have failed to notice or act on indications of encroaching incompetency, and they have not sought an assessment until difficulties have reached a crisis point. Timely and well-planned intervention can certainly reduce the likelihood of a refusal.

When people do refuse to cooperate with an assessment, legal means exist to compel them to accept one, if there are sufficient reasons for doing so. The available means vary from place to place and from case to case. If faced with a person who refuses, but obviously requires, a competency assessment, advice should be sought of a lawyer, state, provincial, or municipal public-health official, or a health-care professional experienced in dealing with incompetent people.

Quite apart from practical considerations, telling someone in advance of a proposed competency assessment is simply the decent and morally correct thing to do. It is also best for the patient. The way that someone is brought for an assessment can impair his or her performance. A competency assessment is a test, and emotionally upset people often have a hard time doing well on any sort of test. Someone who comes to an assessment feeling hurt, betrayed, and coerced is much less likely to perform well on it and thus much more likely to be found incompetent. People should do all that they reasonably can to help others display their best abilities at a competency assessment, and this includes minimizing the emotional upset attendant on the assessment.

Competence and underlying disabilities

When non-specialists assess competency, they generally can do no more than identify tasks that the person cannot perform well. A psychiatrist or other formal assessor will also examine conduct, but in addition will try to identify the particular underlying abilities that the person has lost. Where an untrained observer might know only that someone can no longer fill out checks, for example, a clinical psychologist might determine that the person has the memory and judgment to perform the task but lacks the concentration to do so. Formal assessors, in other words, can sometimes look beneath the surface of incompetence. The light shed by such in-depth assessment can illuminate – for example, it may allow an assessor to devise means of helping a person overcome his or her disabilities. But this light may also blind; there is a tremendous temptation, to which some assessors succumb, to equate disabilities with incompetence. People should never be, but sometimes are, found incompetent only because they suffer from a mental disability. Merely identifying an underlying disability (say, the loss of short-term memory) does not prove that a person is incapable of performing a particular task; the existence of medical or psychological deficiencies and illnesses is not proof of incompetency.

The principal means of assessing mental disabilities that underlie, or are suggestive of, incompetency is psychological testing. The administration of one widely used psychological test, called the Mental State Examination (MSE), will be described in a case example below. Testing is an extremely valuable, and often indispensable, part of most formal competency assessments, but often it is misused. Psychological tests cannot generally prove incompetency, and, in general, people should not be declared incompetent solely on the basis of their performance on such tests.

The first reason why this is so is that proper competency assessment is task-specific and focused on the patient's ability to perform well in the circumstances of his or her own life. But test scores are not always reliable indicators of actual performance. Psychological tests reveal the nature of a person's underlying mental problems, not how these problems actually manifest themselves in the person's life. All that the tests measure is the presence or absence of a set of abilities, but questions of competency cannot be reduced to that level. In fact, the same underlying deficit can render one person incompetent, yet not another person living in different circumstances. Psychological tests are reductionist – they view competency as something much simpler than it really is. Medical and psychological diagnosis is an indispensable part, but still only a part, of competency assessment.

The second reason is that psychological tests lend themselves to false inferences. Some day there may be reliable tests of specific competencies, for example, a test specifically for financial competency, another specifically for competency to make medical decisions, and so on. At present this kind of test does not exist; the reason is that the complex relationship of ability and performance is not yet fully understood. Yet assessors sometimes assume that failure on a psychological test proves the absence of a particular competency. Such conclusions are false inferences, based on the assumption that the abilities tested are the same ones as are needed to be competent to perform a specific task. Only in the clearest of cases is it possible to treat a low test score as conclusive evidence of incompetency, and in such cases the person tested is often so manifestly impaired that the test merely confirms the obvious.

Tests are, however, often legitimately used to *identify* those who are in need of a competency assessment, or to confirm the outcome of an informal competency assessment. Many widely used and reliable psychological tests do give an accurate general picture of an individual's mental state and abilities. Although they cannot prove that a person is incompetent to perform a specific task, they can give important clues that make it easier to assess task-specific competency. Testing can pinpoint a person's strengths and weaknesses and thereby suggest areas, or kinds of tasks, at which he or she is likely to fail; that is, psychological tests alert assessors to the possibility of certain kinds of failures, but do not prove that they will in fact occur. The mere fact that someone has a weak memory, for example, does not prove that he or she is financially incompetent. The knowledge that a person's memory is impaired is at best a starting point from which a thorough assessor would advance to inquire into the complexity of the person's financial affairs (the more complicated they are the more demanding of memory they will be) and into ways of overcoming the impairment (perhaps there is someone who will supply the person with information that he or she cannot retain in memory).

To sum up, psychological tests may help, but alone they do not reveal what people can and cannot do in everyday life.

More than one session needed

The absence of accurate psychological tests of task-specific competence does not render competency assessment imprecise or subjective. Rather, it means that precision and objectivity come only with thoroughness. A valid competency assessment must look at many different aspects of the person and is often quite time-consuming. 'One-shot' assessments that are based on a single meeting with an individual should be viewed with skepticism, except for assessments performed on people, like those in an advanced stage of Alzheimer's disease, who are manifestly and grossly incompetent.

There are many reasons why a proper competency assessment generally cannot be completed in one session. The primary and most common reason for several sessions is that people are nervous at first and need time to become comfortable with the assessor if they are to perform at their best. As well, competency assessments must take account of the whole person and so almost always involve discussions with relatives, friends, or health-care professionals (nurses, social workers, speech therapists, etc.) in addition to discussions with the person being assessed. It is sometimes also necessary to secure a specialized neurological or other medical assessment to rule out the possibility that seemingly incompetent behavior stems from an illness or condition that can be treated medically.

More important, the crucial question in a competency assessment is whether or not a person is capable of making choices. An important (although not always conclusive and certainly not infallible) way of distinguishing choices is by their persistence. Repeated visits are often the only way to determine whether a person persistently expresses the same desires. Finally, with older people, or with people recovering from accidents or illnesses, it is often necessary to keep sessions short lest fatigue masquerade as incompetence. As a general rule one meeting is an insufficient basis for a valid competency assessment. In competency assessment, patience is most definitely a virtue.

Serving the patient's interest

The primary legal and moral obligation of those who perform competency assessments is to serve the person whom they are assessing. On occasion people are brought for a competency assessment by someone who wants to further an immoral or illegal purpose of his or her own.

Although the vast majority of people who challenge another's competency are moved only by a sincere desire to help an ill relative or friend, assessors have a duty to prevent abuse of the assessment process. They should insist on knowing why relatives or friends want to have the person assessed, and in some circumstances they should refuse to perform an assessment until a lawyer has been retained to protect the person being assessed. The relatives and friends who challenge another's competency have a corresponding obligation to accept practices or procedures that may seem insulting, but that are necessary to weed out inappropriate assessment requests. For example, it is fairly common for older people to give real property to a relative because the gift giver can no longer look after it, or as part of estate and tax planning, or for other valid reasons. Often lawyers or family members will seek an assessment of an elderly person's competency to make a gift of real property; such an assessment should not be performed unless the gift giver has his or her own lawyer. Those who seek an assessment on another's behalf should recognize that an assessor's wariness reflects only a justifiable desire to protect patients' rights. Indeed, people should welcome an assessor's inquiries into their motives for seeking an assessment as a positive sign. An assessor who is careful to avoid serving the wrong interest is also likely to be thorough in the assessment.

Which competency is in issue?

A formal competency assessment should never be a fishing expedition for incompetency. Formal assessments invade people's privacy; can often be embarrassing, worrying, or painful; sometimes result in the loss of legal rights; and are expensive and time consuming. A formal assessment should never take place unless there is good reason to believe that it is necessary. 'Necessary' means, among other things, that there is reason to believe that the person to be assessed is at risk of harm because he or she is incompetent to perform a specific task or tasks. It is therefore extremely helpful when an informal assessment of competency has been carried out before a formal one: when the people who seek an assessment are able to specify areas of risk it is much easier to structure a formal assessment properly. Nonetheless, people often seek an assessment without having thought through their reasons for doing so; the assessor must then help them focus and articulate their fears, or must undertake his or her own informal assessment before agreeing to conduct a formal assessment. A formal assessment should, from its outset, focus on task-specific competency, and a careful assessor will therefore require some evidence of specific risk before agreeing to perform an assessment.

The role of friends and family

The first job for family members and friends in a formal assessment of competency is to identify the specific competency that it is in issue. Those who regularly observe a person in daily life are usually well positioned to know what specific tasks he or she may be incompetent to perform. Family and friends must also recognize their own importance. A competency assessor will sometimes determine that a person is competent so long as he or she receives adequate assistance from relatives or friends: on their own they can sometimes render a person competent. For example, Mr L.H. (the man whose children want him to live in a nursing home) was competent to live in the community as long as his daughter was willing and able to care for him, but became incompetent when his daughter was no longer willing and able to do so. This is a particularly clear case because Mr L.H. is so heavily dependent on his daughter. In many other cases, small actions can make a large difference; often, for example, elderly people are capable of functioning in their homes but not outside them; such people can often avoid institutionalization if there is someone to purchase food and other necessities for them.

There are many ways to help people avoid incompetency. Open communication between the relatives and friends of a person who is being assessed and the assessor is almost always helpful and may even be crucial to the performance of a fair and accurate assessment. To some extent this communication may have to be one-way. Legal and moral obligations often prevent an assessor from revealing information about an assessment, even to family and friends. But a professional assessor who is unable to share information should often be willing to receive it. The process of assessment is much fairer, and more accurate, if relatives and friends share their knowledge and experience of the person who is being assessed, and if assessors recognize the value of that information.

Fairness

People may be deprived of their legal rights on the basis of a competency assessment, and assessors therefore have a duty to provide fair assessments. Fairness, in this context, has two principal meanings.

1 A competency assessment should focus on specific tasks that there is good reason to believe the person cannot perform.

2 A competency assessment should allow people to perform at their best.

There are many ways that a competency assessor can either unfairly hinder, or fairly enhance, an individual's performance. The general rule is that an assessment must be designed around the circumstances, character, and needs of the individual who is being assessed; assessors will often have to devise novel assessment techniques or devices that meet the circumstances of individual cases. But some problems or needs appear in many cases. In response to these the Competency Clinic has developed some generally useful assessment methods that are discussed immediately below.

Task-specific competency tests

Since there are no reliable task-specific psychological tests assessors should, whenever possible, seek to assess people in the circumstances under which they actually function. For example, a person's capacity to pay bills should be assessed, if possible, at home, where he or she is comfortable and may take advantage of customary memory aids (say, for example, a list of monthly bills). Sometimes, however, people cannot be tested in the circumstances of their own lives – for example, they may be in hospital. In these cases, assessors must devise their own task-specific tests that replicate, as closely as possible, the actual circumstances in which the individual must function.

There are two major considerations when designing a task-specific test of competency. First, *the test must not be trivial.* For example, in a financial competency case it would make little sense merely to test a person's ability to date checks properly, for in practice very little turns on the ability to date a check. Instead, a meaningful test of financial competency might examine a person's ability to read a bill, locate his or her check book, prepare a valid check in payment of the bill, and then insert the check in a properly addressed envelope for posting.

Second, *the test must be individualized*; it must test the individual's ability to perform tasks in the actual circumstances of his or her own life. For example, it would be unfair to test a person's ability to write a check if that person did not ordinarily pay bills by check; indeed many people pay their bills by automatic withdrawals from their bank accounts. In such a case, a meaningful competency assessment might require a person to review his or her monthly bank statement, explain the meaning of each withdrawal listed on it, and spot any significant errors.

Third, *a fair test must be as realistic as possible.* If someone is asked to fill out a banking form (say a withdrawal slip) the form should come from the bank that the person actually uses. Or, when assessing the ability to make safe use of kitchen appliances it is much better (although not always possible) to watch people in their own kitchens using their own appliances rather than in a hospital kitchen. If an assessment cannot be done in a person's own kitchen an attempt can still be made to replicate the actual circumstances of the person's life; for example, the person's competency could be assessed only with respect to appliances that he or she actually uses. Someone who cooks only with a microwave oven should not be asked to cook on a stove burner. An individual's competence should be judged in the circumstances of his or her own life.

Allowing people to function at their best

Assessors should also be aware that the ability to perform specific tasks can vary significantly at different times. We are all aware that there are days when we do well and others – as after a late night – when our normal standard of performance is unusually difficult. The same is true of people who are being assessed for incompetency.

Fluctuating competency

Some people are competent at some times and incompetent at others. The competency of these people is said to 'fluctuate,' and it is important to distinguish fluctuating competency from incompetency. Too often people whose competency fluctuates are wrongly labelled as incompetent. This error has two common causes. First, the assessment involved only one session, which occurred while the person was incompetent. Second, the assessor did not recognize that intervals of competency are sufficient for some decisions. Fluctuating incompetency does render people incapable of performing some acts, like driving a car, that can be done only by those who are able to make decisions quickly and frequently. But many tasks require only that a person be competent when issuing instructions or making other decisions. For example, a valid will may sometimes be made during a period of lucidity by a person who is at other times incompetent. In other circumstances a person whose competency fluctuates but who is aware of a specific problem may well be competent to decide on it. Consider, for example, a person whose competency fluctuates but who while competent persistently expresses a wish to continue living in her own apartment as opposed to a nursing home. If this woman also recognizes the peculiar risks to which her periodic incompetency may expose her – that is, if while competent she recognizes that she is not always so – she is capable of deciding where she will reside.

As a general rule a person whose competency fluctuates, but who expresses the same desire or wish during at least two intervals of competency, is competent. A useful way to describe such people is to say that their competency fluctuates but their wishes or decisions are persistent and consistent; these people express the same wish over time during periods of competency that are separated by periods of incompetency.

Fluctuating competency is particulary common in elderly people whose level of alertness varies dramatically throughout the day. It is important to assess elderly or frail individuals' ability to make particular decisions at the time of day when they are usually at their best. An assessor who suspects that a person's competence fluctuates will, in the absence of information from relatives, friends, or health-care providers, often have to perform repeated assessments until he or she hits on the time of day when the person is at his or her best.

There is another useful rule that should be applied when a person need be competent only when issuing an instruction or performing a particular act. In such cases the assessment should be performed while, or shortly before, the act is performed or the instruction is issued; in many cases (particularly when someone is giving instructions for the preparation of a will or is executing one) the assessor becomes a disinterested witness to the person's competency. When assessing competency to issue an instruction or to perform an act, testing should often be both task- and time-specific.

Temporary incompetence

People may also be rendered temporarily incompetent by an illness or accident. It is therefore sometimes desirable to delay an assessment in the hope that the person's incompetency will abate, if the delay is legally permissible and is not too risky (as it might be, for example, if the patient's financial affairs require immediate attention). People, especially older people, are often disoriented when they are taken to hospital following an accident or medical emergency. It is only fair to wait until such people have become accustomed to their new surroundings and have come to terms with any damage they have suffered before assessing them. As well, assessors should always learn about any medications or drugs that people are taking and (if possible) avoid assessing them while they are under the influence of any substance that impairs mental function. If a person's incompetence may be temporary, but an assessment cannot be delayed, an assessor who wishes to be fair may still proceed with the assessment, but will schedule a reassessment for a later time.

Competency assessments should not create failure

A poorly executed competency assessment can actually cause a competent person to appear incompetent. One frequent cause of poor performance at an assessment is nervousness. Many people perform poorly under pressure, particularly if they are used to living an undemanding life. If an assessor suspects that a person is performing poorly because of nervousness, there are two remedies to consider; the assessment can be temporarily interrupted while the assessor tries to calm the overwrought person, or the session can be ended and rescheduled. Another frequent cause of poor performance by older people is the discomfort or disorientation produced by unfamiliar surroundings. Often it is best to assess people, and especially elderly people, in their own homes. A fair competency assessment is designed to impose the least possible stress on the person undergoing assessment.

Correct reasoning versus correct answers

Sometimes a person performs much below his or her apparent capacity at an assessment, most commonly by providing seemingly irrational or incorrect responses to an assessor's questions. In such cases it is often helpful to shift focus from the individual's incorrect answers to his or her reasoning; for example, an assessor might, without saying that an answer may be incorrect, ask a person to explain the reason for the answer given. It is quite common for such questions to reveal that the assessor has failed to grasp the assessed person's reasoning.

For example, Mr F.C. (the man who had a stroke and who now wishes to regain control of his financial affairs) says that he will sell a number of his possessions if he regains control of his finances. The assessor therefore tests Mr F.C.'s ability to conduct a sale. She asks him to describe how he would sell an antique pendant that he wants to dispose of. Mr F.C. proposes to place an advertisement in an antique collector's newsletter offering the pendant for sale at a price of $8,000. Earlier, Mr F.C. had told the assessor that the pendant has an appraised value of $15,000. It seems to the assessor that Mr F.C.'s proposal is irrational, and this contradicts her general impression of him as an alert and thoughtful person, so she asks Mr F.C. how he arrived at the figure of $8,000. He replies that jewellery generally sells at a substantial discount from its appraised value, and that $8,000 is probably about $500 above the pendant's actual market value. Mr F.C.'s seemingly incorrect answer was actually quite sensible, but only to someone who knows about the market for antique jewelry. It is important not to conclude that a person is incompetent simply because some of his or her answers appear to be incorrect.

There is a further reason for examining the quality of a person's reasoning: seemingly incorrect answers may disclose defects in the test or testing process. A question that seems very straightforward to the examiner may be ambiguous to the person tested. In such a case what appears to be an incorrect answer may actually be a sensible reply to an interpretation of the question that differs from the assessor's intended meaning.

Physical disabilities, such as bad hearing or poor eyesight, may also prevent a competent person from properly comprehending a test or question. A careful assessor therefore treats each assessment as an investigation not only of the subject's competency but also of the validity of the tests and testing procedures. A careful assessor will always remain open to the possibility that seemingly wrong answers grow out of defects in the test or testing process.

Choosing the right assessor

A competency assessment involves asking people to open their lives up to others' scrutiny. Some people are simply uncomfortable talking about personal matters. Others may be willing to do so, but not with the members of the opposite sex (or, in other cases, of the same sex); in such cases, the gender of the assessor should be considered carefully. However strongly an assessor believes in gender equality, he or she should, in the interest of obtaining a fair and thorough assessment, strive to recognize and accommodate the subject's own preferences and feelings. Assessors must pay careful attention to the *kind* of person whom they are assessing.

Asking tough and upsetting questions

As important as it is to make people feel comfortable during a competency assessment, it is also sometimes impossible – and unfair – to avoid asking them tough and upsetting questions. Ordinarily, if a friend or relative has a wrong idea about something, people tell them so; indeed, correcting another's errors is a form of respect. Correcting another's mistake implies that the person both can and wants to correct his or her errors, that is, is capable of learning. Refusing to point out errors to a person amounts to a presumption of incompetence, namely, that the person is incapable of recognizing and correcting errors. Moreover, by not challenging apparent mistakes assessors deprive the person being assessed of the opportunity to prove that it is the assessor who has fallen into error (as with Mr F.C. whose reasoning was not wrong, only based on a better knowledge of the antique jewelry market than his assessor had).

Furthermore, if a person's competency is challenged because of specific mistakes that he or she has made (or is likely to make) it is only fair to tell him or her so. That provides an opportunity for the person to explain the questionable conduct or to consider means of coming to terms with an obvious incompetency. Sometimes (as with a person who makes glaring errors during an assessment, such as writing the wrong amount on checks) a tough question may confront a person with unassailable evidence of his or her incompetence. The risk of asking hard questions is that they may confuse or demoralize an incompetent person. The risk of not asking hard questions is that the failure to do so, although well motivated, denies the person a fair opportunity to display his or her real abilities.

Only good judgment and experience can determine when a confrontational question has gone too far. As a rule of thumb it is preferable to err in favour of giving people the fullest reasonable opportunity to display their abilities. Family and friends should not be upset at tough and upsetting questions from a competency assessor. They should consider *before* seeking a formal competency assessment that it may be a hurtful experience, because a fair assessment is sometimes necessarily an upsetting one.

Incompetence vs. ignorance

A competency assessment can often become an exercise in devising ways to make it possible for the subject to be judged competent. An assessment sometimes reveals, for example, that a person who appears to be incompetent may simply lack the information that he or she needs to make decisions. For instance, a person may need to arrange his finances but have no experience with financial matters; or, a person may want someone else to handle her financial affairs but be unaware of the means by which she may choose her own financial substitute decision maker. In cases where a person appears to lack relevant information an assessor should generally suspend the assessment and refer the person to an appropriate adviser. People cannot be expected to manage competently matters or decisions that they do not understand; sometimes only after an individual has been provided with appropriate information may his or her competency be accurately assessed.

Memory loss can also make a person who is capable of making decisions seem to be incapable of doing so. Some memory-impaired people are quite able to make decisions, but only if someone else provides them with information that they cannot hold in their own minds. For example, Mr F.C. (the man who has recovered from a stroke and wishes to regain control of his financial affairs) clearly has moderately impaired short- and long-term memory. His psychiatrist fears that if Mr F.C. regains control of his financial affairs he will forget to do important things and thereby suffer financial losses. The psychiatrist tells Mr F.C. of his fear, challenges him to find a solution to his problem, and actually gives Mr F.C. his assignment in writing so that he will not forget it. At his next meeting with the psychiatrist Mr F.C. appears with a list of his major assets that his bookkeeper has prepared for him. The psychiatrist reviews the list with Mr F.C. who is able to explain, in some detail, what each item is and what he proposes to do with it if he regains control of his finances. Mr F.C. proposes to sell most of his assets and invest the proceeds in a small number of bonds and blue chip stocks. Mr F.C.'s bookkeeper will prepare a monthly list of all his financial holdings and will maintain a list of the dividends that he should receive from his stocks and bonds. Mr F.C. has also purchased a diary in which he will record every task that he must perform (for example, depositing dividend checks in the bank). The psychiatrist has a social worker speak to Mr F.C.'s bookkeeper to confirm that she is indeed willing to provide the assistance that Mr F.C. wants. The psychiatrist now knows that despite his memory loss Mr F.C. is capable of exercising financial judgment and of directing others in the execution of tasks that he cannot perform himself. For Mr F.C. assessment has become a means of restoring his competence. A competency assessment may reveal both a person's underlying problem and the means of overcoming it.

Communication

People who have had a stroke, or who have suffered a brain injury, often lose their ability to speak, or to write, or both. With modern technology, including computers, specialized assistance (often from a speech therapist, a health-care professional who specializes in diagnosing and correcting speech problems), and time, even extremely impaired people may learn to communicate at a very high level. Assessing the competency of people who use speech aids is more time-consuming, but otherwise little different from assessing the competency of a person who can speak.

There are many cases where someone's competency (usually to make a decision about medical treatment) is in question and an assessment must be conducted quickly; in these circumstances there is often no time to consult with a speech therapist or to use sophisticated speech aids. As well, there is often no money to do either. But the inability to verbalize, even if specialized help is unavailable, does not always mean that a person cannot communicate at all. With a little originality, crude but reliable communication, sufficient for the purposes of a competency assessment, can be established even with extremely disabled people; an example of such an assessment is included in this chapter.

There are also a range of less serious failures of communication that can, if undetected, impair the fairness or accuracy of an assessment. One common problem in contemporary multicultural societies is the assessment of people who can speak, but are not fluent in, the languages most commonly used. It is easy enough to detect someone who speaks no, or very little, English, French, or Spanish, but it is harder to detect people who speak a common language well enough to get by most of the time, but not well enough to explain their reasoning or priorities in life, as people must often do in a competency assessment. To make certain that lack of fluency is not confused with incompetency, an assessor should ask the family what language the person being assessed speaks most comfortably. If it seems desirable, assessment should be conducted with the assistance of an interpreter. A family member may sometimes provide interpretation, but it is much preferable to obtain the services of a disinterested person if possible.

Another problem that may affect ability to communicate – one that is quite common among older people – is loss of hearing. If the person being assessed accepts the existence of an impairment and takes steps to overcome it (which may mean no more than asking the assessor to speak slowly, distinctly, and loudly), hearing loss may do little more than slow the pace of the assessment. But it is not uncommon for people to deny that they are becoming hard of hearing and to refuse to wear a hearing aid, even though they cannot hear reliably without one. An assessor who suspects that a person suffers from an unacknowledged or unrevealed hearing problem should ask the person's family doctor, relatives, or friends whether there is a hearing problem which might hinder the assessment. If someone does have impaired hearing but refuses to take steps to remedy the problem, the assessment may still proceed, but the assessor must be careful to establish reliable communication. In some instances this may require no more than sitting at a reasonable distance from the person so that he or she can comfortably read lips, or speaking more slowly and distinctly than normal. In more extreme instances the assessment may be conducted in writing. Finally, in some cases a refusal to accept and accommodate a hearing loss may indicate that the person is incompetent, and it is certainly an item for concern if the person's ability to conduct his or her day-to-day affairs is in issue.

Medical or psychiatric illness

The assessment of people suffering from major mental illnesses like schizophrenia or severe depression can pose peculiar difficulties. Indeed, a book could be written on this subject alone. There are, however, some common problems that merit inclusion even in a general book like this.

The most difficult cases are those in which it is hard to know whether a person's desires are an expression of beliefs and preferences (that is, a choice) or merely a reflection of an illness. For example, when someone who is depressed refuses a medical treatment that may prolong his or her life but will be quite painful, it is hard to know whether that person has rationally weighed the benefit of treatment against the cost of pain, or whether the hopelessness engendered by depression has led to passive and irrational acceptance of an avoidable death. People are often tempted to resolve such cases simply by asking whether they might, if in the shoes of a person with a major mental illness, make the same decision as that person has. But the fact that a person's decision is comprehensible to others does not alone make that person competent; a test of empathy or reasonableness which assumes that the assessor's and the assessed's preferences and beliefs are the same actually invites undue paternalism. In short, such an approach is a cop-out – a refusal by the assessor to face up to the real difficulties involved in determining whether the person being assessed is capable of making choices.

A better approach to assessing someone suffering from a major mental illness is to have an experienced professional evaluate the nature and severity of the illness and compare the person's wishes, goals, or preferences with those that he or she held when well. The assessment of people whose illness or disability is unrelenting (as, for example, with those schizophrenics who are almost constantly ill and do not respond to treatment) can be extremely difficult, however, for in such cases there is no state of wellness against which the effects of illness may be assessed. Similar problems may be encountered when assessing the functional competency of a person who has spent a large part of his or her adult life in institutions. In such cases it may be impossible to distinguish inexperience from incompetency, and the assessment may in fairness have to focus on the person's capacity either to master new and unfamiliar skills or to select appropriate assistants, rather than on his or her present functioning. In some cases of extremely severe illness it is reasonable to depart from the general rule that prohibits inferring incompetency from the presence of illness, and to conclude that the very severe illness (without further functional testing) is evidence of incompetence; but this approach should be adopted only as a last resort and only in very clear cases.

Three competency assessments

Following these general principles is not always easy. By returning to three of the fictional cases introduced in chapter 1, we can see how the principles may be applied to provide thorough and fair competency assessments. The first case demonstrates the use of a general psychological test, to present a clear picture of what these tests are and of the kind of valuable information they can yield. The particular test demonstrated is the Mental State Examination, and it is applied to an assessment of financial competency. The second case demonstrates the performance of a team assessment, to show how members of different disciplines may approach competency assessment. This case approximates the performance of a team assessment in the Competency Clinic at the Baycrest Centre for Geriatric Care. The third case involves the assessment of a person who can neither speak nor write, and it shows how ingenuity and concern may sometimes overcome grave difficulties in communication.

Mr F.C. ten years on: Financial competency and the Mental Status Examination

Mr F.C. is the man whose memory was moderately impaired by a stroke, but who nonetheless devised a plan that restored him to financial competency. Ten years have passed since Mr F.C. regained control of his financial affairs; he is now seventy-five and fate has been unkind to him. Five years ago his wife died. Following her death he had a series of small strokes. Mr F.C. has a grandson who is an accountant and also has Mr F.C.'s absolute trust. The grandson has recently begun to suspect that Mr F.C. is no longer competent to manage his own finances. He discusses his fears with his brother and with Mr F.C.'s general practitioner, who share them. The doctor refers Mr F.C. to a psychiatrist for an assessment of his financial competency.

What is financial competency?

Financial competency consists of the ability to make considered decisions regarding financial matters, combined with the instrumental abilities needed to execute those decisions. Instrumental abilities include literacy, memory, and a suitable understanding of numbers. Their mere absence does not alone make a person financially incompetent: people may be deprived by illness, disease, or age of some instrumental ability but retain the capacity to oversee someone else (for example, a bookkeeper) who executes their decisions for them. An assessment of financial competency thus must usually canvass at least three significant and distinct elements.

1 The person's own considered or habitual views of and approaches to financial matters;

2 The circumstances in which the person actually makes decisions; and,

3 The complexity of the financial affairs concerned.

For example, a man who has always been cavalier about financial matters – who is somewhat eccentric in such matters – is not incompetent simply because he continues a lifelong pattern of financial sloppiness. The same man might well be determined incompetent, however, if he had recently lost the ability to work, was now totally dependent on a small pension, and was incapable of appreciating the new risks associated with his sloppiness. As well, the degree of ability required to make and execute financial decisions will depend on the complexity of a person's financial affairs. Thus, someone whose finances are very straightforward may well be financially competent, although the same person would be incapable of making decisions regarding very complicated and sophisticated financial matters. A person might be competent to manage a small pension income, but incompetent to manage a sizeable and diverse portfolio of stocks and bonds. In sum, financially competent people have the ability to dispose of their money and property in accordance with their habitual or considered standards and with an awareness of the likely consequences of the decisions that they make.

Visiting the psychiatrist

Mr F.C. and his grandson have a frank discussion of the grandson's fear that Mr F.C. can no longer independently manage his financial affairs. The grandson assures his grandfather of his love and his desire to help him, but says that he cannot help without knowing exactly what his grandfather's problems are. He then asks Mr F.C. to meet with a psychiatrist for the purpose of a competency assessment. The grandfather consents. The grandson takes Mr F.C. to his first meeting with the psychiatrist and introduces Mr F.C. to her. She asks the grandson, in Mr F.C.'s presence, to explain why he thinks an assessment is necessary. He replies that he thinks his grandfather is no longer financially competent, but that he (the grandson) is willing to become his attorney or guardian. The psychiatrist is not satisfied with this explanation and wants to know about specific instances where Mr F.C. has failed to perform financial tasks adequately. The grandson tells her of Mr F.C.'s medical history and describes some recent events that suggest that Mr F.C. may be incompetent. Mr F.C. forgot to pay several large bills; he threw away some dividend checks thinking that they were receipts; he neglected to cash thousands of dollars in matured Canada Savings Bonds that were in his safety deposit box, thus losing a considerable amount of interest. The psychiatrist notes all these incidents (and the grandson's willingness to help his grandfather) and then asks the grandson to leave her alone with Mr F.C. The psychiatrist intends to ask Mr F.C. for his version of events, and it would be an invasion of his privacy to ask him to do so in the presence of a relative. She also wishes to show him that she respects, and will protect, his right to privacy.

After the grandson leaves the room the psychiatrist asks Mr F.C. what he has to say about the events that his grandson described. Mr F.C. does not remember any of them, and he simply says that he sometimes becomes very tired and finds things confusing. Mr F.C. is by now visibly anxious and upset. At this point in the interview the psychiatrist decides that she has enough information to justify assessing Mr F.C.'s financial competency.

She calms Mr F.C., explaining that many older people find they need some help to do things they used to do themselves and it is quite natural for someone who has had a series of strokes to experience confusion and fatigue. She will, she tells Mr F.C., do everything she can to help him, and she would like to perform some tests on him that may reveal the kind of help that he needs. She also tells him that she can do these tests only if he wants to have them done and that he has every right to refuse them. Furthermore, she explains, as a result of the tests she may conclude that he is incompetent and her conclusion might cause someone to apply to become his guardian. She asks Mr F.C. to explain to her what he thinks guardianship entails, and he tells her that it would mean that he would be unable to make his own financial decisions. She then asks him whether he understands that if he agrees to be tested he could well lose control of his finances. He says that he understands this, but he wants to know what is 'going on with him' and would like her to do the tests. Satisfied that she has her patient's consent, the psychiatrist begins the formal assessment.

The psychiatrist customarily begins her assessments by administering a psychological test called the Mental Status Examination (hereafter MSE). Had she not already requested that the grandson leave her alone with Mr F.C., she would certainly have done so at this point. She generally will not administer a psychological test with third parties present unless her patient asks that they remain. A psychological test can reveal intimate and embarrassing matters, and people are as entitled to have it administered in private as they are to have physical examinations that require them to disrobe administered in private.

The Mental Status Examination

The MSE is a test of thought processes, emotions, feelings, and mood used by assessors to form a general impression of an individual. The components of the test evaluate mood; perception and involuntary or unconscious difficulties that affect it; orientation to time, place, and person; memory; and social judgment. Many other tests are also some-times used in competency assessment, among them the Cognitive Competency Test, the Mini-Mental Status Examination, the Competency Decisional Aid (a test developed at the Competency Clinic of the

Baycrest Centre for Geriatric Care). A variety of other instruments have been devised specifically for use with elderly people or on those who are suspected to be suffering from a dementia of some kind.

The first part of the test assesses *mood.* Here the assessor is primarily looking for emotions and feelings that may adversely affect the individual's judgment and for emotional states that point to the existence of deeper mental problems. The assessor must decide what the person's mood is (elated, anxious, sad, etc.); whether the person's mood fluctuates during the interview (extreme and inappropriate mood changes are symptoms of a number of deeper problems); and whether the person's appearance and behavior are consistent with his or her mood. As well, the assessor is looking for any disparity between the person's own (that is, subjective) assessment of his or her mood and the objective evidence of mood supplied by a careful assessment of the person's appearance. Mr F.C.'s mood is somewhat despondent, which is quite natural for someone who has just been confronted with evidence of his failing mental abilities. However, the psychiatrist notes that Mr F.C's mood changes erratically throughout the interview and that he is given to emotional extremes. In technical terms, Mr F.C. is emotionally labile (unstable), a state that is sometimes indicative of a deeper mental problem.

Another part of the test examines the *content and flow of the person's thoughts.* The assessor will try to elicit the kinds of thoughts that currently preoccupy the person being assessed. For example, a person who is preoccupied with thoughts of suicide may well be suffering from depression. As well, the assessor will try to determine during this part of the test whether a person is suffering from delusions. A delusion is an unusual or inexplicable belief that has no basis in fact and that no amount of rational disproof can persuade the person to abandon. A person may possess an intractable belief, say, that the police are sending death rays through his television set. Finally, the assessor will look for evidence of disruption in the stream of sequence of thought, rather than in its content. Here the assessor looks to see how the person's thoughts relate one to the next, for disconnected or erratic thoughts are indicative of some kinds of mental illness. The conversation of some mentally ill people, for example, meanders disjointedly from topic to topic without apparent coherence, direction, or plan, and they may, when questioned, be unable to retrace their own mental steps. Mr F.C.'s responses in this part of the test reveal no abnormality in his thought processes.

A third part studies the patient's *perception and vegetative symptoms.* Perception is the ability to see, hear, and feel. Most individuals' senses react only to external stimuli; they see a car drive past them, hear their spouses call their name, or feel their cats rubbing against their legs. But sometimes people see, hear, or feel things that are not actually present, without any rational or plausible explanation for their perceptions; this kind of false or disordered perception is called hallucination. Hallucinations are commonly either visual (the person has visions of things that are not present) or auditory (the person hears voices, but no one is talking). Hallucinations are often symptoms of mental illness, although they can also result from some medications or from the consumption of alcohol or drugs.

Vegetative symptoms relate to basic biological processes like eating, sleeping, thinking, and movement. Marked alterations in some or all of these basic processes are sometimes indicative of mental illness, such as severe depression. To reveal any vegetative symptoms the assessor asks questions about such things as appetite, sleep habits, energy level, and the pace of the person's movement or thought. Again, Mr F.C.'s answers to questions about his perceptions and vegetative symptoms suggest nothing at all abnormal.

The questions in the next part relate to *orientation in space and time.* They seek to determine whether the person recognizes where he or she is; is able to explain how he or she got there; is aware of the time, date, and season; knows who he or she is; and is capable of recognizing people who play a significant role in his or her life (for example, a spouse). Questions about orientation are particularly likely to identify people who have a dementia or who have suffered brain damage, as Mr F.C. has. People in an advanced stage of dementia, or who have suffered grave brain injuries, often are unable to give the correct time, date, or season; they may not know where they are, and they may even be unable to identify themselves correctly. Mr F.C. knows who he is and that he is in a psychiatrist's office, but he is not sure where the office is. He cannot remember how he got there. He knows what time it is, but not the date or the season. Mr F.C.'s answers suggest that he has some kind of underlying mental disability.

The MSE also examines *memory* – generally divided into three categories: immediate, recent, and long term. As a test of immediate memory, the person is given a task that requires ongoing attention and concentration. A typical assignment is called 'serial sevens'; in this test the examiner asks the person to subtract 7 from 100 until the balance is 0; usually the test stops after the subject has performed the task successfully three to five times). The task requires the person to keep in mind the number to be subtracted (7) and also the number from which 7 must now be subtracted. To test recent memory, the person is asked to memorize a series of words and then, a short time later (say ten minutes), to recall them. This task examines the person's ability to retain new information, and so to learn. Finally, questions about the person's past are used to examine long-term memory. For example, a person may be questioned about old addresses, or telephone numbers.

Memory disorders have various and complex consequences. Some people with memory disorders have an excellent knowledge of their past but are unable to retain new information, that is, to learn. Other people have a very poor knowledge of their past yet are able to retain new information. Sometimes the attention and concentration of people with advanced dementias, or severe brain damage, is so poor that it is possible to test only their immediate memory.

Mr F.C. has very poor long-term memory, recalls only one of the four words that he was asked to memorize, and has to be continually prompted to continue subtracting 7; even with prompting he does the subtraction only twice before abandoning it. Thinking that the problem might lie in the size of the number, the psychiatrist asks him to try the test using 3 instead of 7, but the result is little different. Mr F.C.'s results suggest that his memory is impaired in all three categories and that his ability to learn is probably quite limited.

One final section of the test examines *social judgment*. The person is asked to imagine how he or she might respond in a hypothetical social situation. For example, the assessor might say: 'You are shopping in a large department store, and someone yells, "Fire!" What would you do?' This part of the test is also used to determine whether the person being assessed has a realistic understanding of his or her own circumstances; the assessor might also ask: 'What would you do if a fire broke out in your own home?' Mr F.C.'s answers to these questions generally display a lack of good social judgment, although he does seem to recognize that some of his mental abilities have become impaired and that he is no longer able to do some things that he used to be able to do. His responses are at times unusual; for example, when asked what he would do if his house caught fire he replies, 'Watch it burn.' The psychiatrist wonders whether Mr F.C. has lost, perhaps as a consequence of brain damage caused by his strokes, some of the inhibitions that ordinarily restrain his behavior.

Interpreting the test

Mr F.C.'s psychiatrist is well aware that the MSE is designed to reveal and diagnose underlying mental disorders and that it is not a test of task-specific competency; she therefore does not conclude that he is financially incompetent only because of his poor test performance. However, the test results confirm her opinion that there is good reason to assess Mr F.C.'s financial competency; she also now wants him to have a thorough medical and neurological examination that she hopes will reveal the cause of his problems. She also has some ideas about the kinds of financial tasks that he may have difficulty performing. The particular areas that concern her are his ability to remember, on an ongoing basis, financial tasks that he has to perform; his ability to concentrate long enough to perform tasks that involve manipulating numbers; his ability to remember what he is doing long enough to complete any task that takes more than a minute or so to complete; and, finally, his ability to make choices. Her fear on this last point is that Mr F.C. may tend to act impulsively and so expose himself to the risk of financial loss. The psychiatrist also wants to know more about how Mr F.C. has actually been conducting his finances. The MSE shows a substantial degree of impairment, and she suspects that either Mr F.C. has made financial mistakes or is receiving assistance that his grandson is unaware of. The psychiatrist particularly hopes that Mr F.C. has already found ways to cope with his disabilities, for this would be powerful evidence that he is financially competent. People who recognize, and make appropriate arrangements to overcome, mental disabilities that affect their financial competency are not financially incompetent.

As well, even if Mr F.C. is financially incompetent he may still be competent to choose his own financial substitute decision maker. Further, the psychiatrist must know more about Mr F.C.'s finances if she is to administer task-specific tests of his financial abilities. In particular she must understand how complex Mr F.C.'s finances are; the precise tasks that he is unable to perform well; whether he is willing to accept help; and whether others are willing to supply the help that he needs. She also wants to interview Mr F.C. in his home, thus eliminating the possibility that his performance in her office was impaired by any disorientation or discomfort that he felt in an unfamiliar environment. A home interview will reveal whether he is able to perform better in a familiar setting and also whether he relies on aids (like a diary) that he would not have available if assessed in her office. Mr F.C. agrees to accept a home visit, and he gives the psychiatrist permission to seek more information about his finances from his grandson.

The home interview

The psychiatrist prepares for her visit with Mr F.C. by speaking with his grandson about Mr F.C.'s finances. She also prepares some financial tests that are closely related to the financial tasks that Mr F.C. actually performs. At the interview she begins by asking Mr F.C. to describe his income and expenses. He produces a list of his assets (somewhat out of date) that his bookkeeper has prepared for him. He is unable to explain what some of the items on the list are. He does not know – even approximately – how much he spends monthly on his expenses or even what they are. Although he recalls that he pays bills for electricity, gas, and telephone he does not mention five other bills that he pays monthly. The psychiatrist then slowly recites aloud a list of common expenses, including all those that Mr F.C. does pay for monthly, hoping that in this way that she will prompt his memory. Indeed, after listening to her he recalls that he pays for cable television and newspaper delivery. The psychiatrist then tells him that he pays for a number of other items, among them groceries delivered by a local store and house cleaning; he replies that he does not know anything about such bills.

The psychiatrist then asks him to make out checks to pay for gas and telephone bills that he has received. She has with her checks of the kind that Mr F.C. ordinarily uses. He gets the amount wrong on one check, and on the other there is a discrepancy between the number that he has expressed in figures ($129.87) and the number that he has expressed in writing (two hundred and twenty-nine dollars and eighty-seven cents). When asked to review the checks he sees nothing wrong with them. When told that they contain errors he is unable to spot them. He is asked where he keeps his stocks and bonds; he answers that they are at his bank, but he cannot recall where his bank is. He is asked how he tells whether he has received, and deposited, the correct number of dividend checks every month, and he cannot answer the question. Finally, the psychiatrist asks Mr F.C. whether anyone has been helping him with his finances; he replies that his bookkeeper gives him a great deal of help. At this point in the interview Mr F.C. is extremely frustrated and very anxious. The psychiatrist decides that it would be wrong to continue the assessment any further at this point. Instead, she sits and chats with Mr F.C. for half an hour, long enough for him to recover his composure.

Mr F.C.'s bookkeeper

With Mr F.C.'s permission the psychiatrist interviews his bookkeeper, and the reason for his recent financial failures becomes evident. Mr F.C.'s bookkeeper has been helping him with many aspects of his finances. She has maintained a list of maturing bonds and expected dividends. She drives him to the bank to pay his bills and retrieve items from his safety deposit box. She also has been making out the checks to pay his bills. She charges him a modest fee for all her work. About six weeks ago, while they were at the bank, he accused her of stealing from him; a number of people, including several tellers and the assistant bank manager, heard the accusation, which Mr F.C.'s grandson later investigated and discovered to be completely unfounded. The bookkeeper was mortified; she has a genuine affection for Mr F.C. and his accusation deeply hurt her. As well, she could not afford to have her integrity challenged in this way; she feared that if Mr F.C. continued with his allegations her other clients would hear that she was cheating a helpless old man. She drove Mr F.C. home, then told him she was unprepared to continue helping him. He said that he would find another bookkeeper, and she has been waiting for someone to collect his financial records from her. Mr F.C. forgot about their fight and her resignation. Without his bookkeeper's help, his financial incompetency revealed itself.

Conclusion

The neurological assessment confirms that Mr F.C. has sustained fairly extensive brain damage. This damage probably explains his uncharacteristic behavior with the bookkeeper. The psychiatrist assesses Mr F.C. at home one more time, with similar results. All the evidence points inescapably to the conclusion that Mr F.C. is financially incompetent. However, the psychiatrist recognizes that for a very long time Mr F.C. was willing to accept help from his bookkeeper, and she seems to have been a really good person to look to for help. The psychiatrist therefore proposes to conduct an assessment of Mr F.C.'s ability to execute a power of attorney. She hopes he has retained the ability to choose an appropriate person to look after his finances; if he has, both Mr F.C. and his grandson may be able to avoid the expense and humiliation of an application to have Mr F.C. declared financially incompetent and his grandson appointed as his guardian. As well, the psychiatrist thinks that this is the least-restrictive alternative course of action open to her, in that it gives Mr F.C. the maximum realistic opportunity to make and act on his own decisions.

Ms M.R.: A multidisciplinary assessment of competency to choose a place of residence

Ms M.R. (the diabetic woman who had a stroke) in the past has lived alone and has successfully monitored and adjusted her diet and use of insulin. Her physicians claim that her stroke has now deprived her of the ability to continue living independently, but she thinks they are wrong and wants to return home as soon as possible. Psychological testing has shown that Ms M.R.'s memory and concentration are impaired. It is not yet possible to tell whether, or to what extent, her memory and concentration will recover. Ms M.R. is referred to a hospital psychiatrist for a competency assessment, to which she consents. Ms M.R. thinks that she will be found competent and will return to her own home. Her physicians think that she will not. They expect that her niece, who is actively involved in Ms M.R.'s care, will apply to become her guardian if Ms M.R. persists in her refusal to accept some kind of institutional home. On reviewing the hospital records, the psychiatrist decides that this case is difficult enough to merit referral to a multidisciplinary competency team that he leads.

The team

The members of the competency team are the psychiatrist, Martin Smith; a social worker, Jack Czerneski; a nurse practitioner, Harriet Campbell; and Brigitte Canning, a medical ethicist who teaches in the philosophy department of a local university.

A social worker who practices in a health-care setting performs several functions; these include helping patients who have chronic medical problems plan for their return to life in the community, providing various kinds of individual and family counselling (depending on local laws and policies and on the social worker's training), and helping people identify and gain access to various kinds of concrete assistance, such as programs that provide in-home services to the elderly. Jack Czerneski holds a master's degree in social work and specializes in helping people with neurological disabilities, and their families, develop reasonable plans for community-based (as opposed to institutional) care. Nurse practitioners are registered nurses who have received training beyond that of ordinary registered nurses and may (again depending on local laws and policies) provide services that ordinary registered nurses do not. Harriet Campbell specializes in dealing with the psychiatrically ill, and she often works with the psychiatrist who leads the assessment team. A medical ethicist (sometimes also called a bioethicist) brings professional training or experience to the consideration and resolution of the sometimes profound moral dilemmas that arise in the provision of medical treatment or other personal care or in connection with research studies. Medical ethicists come from many different professional backgrounds, including law, philosophy, theology, and various areas of health care.

In the performance of assessments Martin Smith and Harriet Campbell usually meet with the patient and the patient's professional caregivers. Jack Czerneski usually meets with the patient's relatives and friends (although Harriet Campbell may also do this). Brigitte Canning never meets with the patients that the team assesses, nor with the patient's relatives and friends. Clinical ethicists often do meet with patients. However, this team finds it advantageous to have one member who is free from the direct emotional bonds and responses (and particularly the desire to protect an obviously frail or vulnerable person) that sometimes distort competency assessments. Moreover, Brigitte herself is content to play this role.

Meeting 1: Necessity

A meeting is convened before which Martin Smith has circulated a brief note to the other members of the team:

Ms M.R. is a 63-year-old woman who is diabetic and who has recently suffered a stroke. It is too early to tell how full a recovery she will stage. Psychological testing has placed her at the threshold of dementia, i.e., her memory and concentration are moderately impaired. Her health-care providers think that she is incapable of caring for herself at home and that a guardianship application is in order if she insists on returning home against medical advice. I have spoken with her, explained what the team is, and she has consented to an assessment. My question is whether we have established necessity for an assessment.

Along with this note are circulated copies of Ms M.R.'s hospital record and of a report from the psychologist who administered tests to her.

The first person to speak at the meeting is the ethicist, Brigitte Canning. Brigitte tends to take a harder line on protecting individual liberty than the other team members do. In part, this is because Brigitte genuinely thinks that it is healthy to maintain a constant tension between the desire to help (a desire felt more powerfully by those who actually meet with the patients) and the obligation to safeguard individual liberty, and in part this is because Brigitte thinks that her role on the team is to act as a devil's advocate. Brigitte's opening comment is typically brusque, 'This woman did well on her own before, and no one can prove that she won't now. All we have is speculation. This is medical paternalism – I say there's no necessity for this assessment.'

Harriet, who has actually met Ms M.R., responds, 'Ms M.R. is really a bad diabetic – if she messes up on her insulin or her diet she could kill herself. Many diabetics have a hard time monitoring their drugs and diet, let alone a woman whose memory and concentration are shaky. *You* should try living your life as carefully as she'll have to live hers. I'm not saying that she's incompetent, but there are strong reasons to fear for her safety.'

Jack agrees with Harriet, but raises a different concern: 'Ms M.R. is just coming back from her stroke, and we should wait [to assess her] until she has recovered.'

Martin Smith asks rhetorically, 'Are you saying that we should keep this woman in the hospital just because she hasn't yet recovered fully? She wants to go home *now*, and if she can there's no reason to hold her in the hospital. Besides, if she's incompetent now, we can reassess her later.'

At the end of the meeting, Brigitte Canning agrees with the others that there is necessity for an assessment of Ms M.R. Collectively they agree that it is in Ms M.R.'s interest to perform the assessment as quickly as possible. The team also sets an agenda for its next meeting. Brigitte is to formulate a working definition of competency to choose place of residence. Harriet is to interview Ms M.R. and the medical staff to get some idea of Ms M.R.'s own thoughts, values, and plans, and to learn more about the regime of diet and medication that Ms M.R. must follow to maintain her health. Jack is to interview Ms M.R.'s niece (if Ms M.R. agrees to allow him to) to see how much support she is prepared to offer Ms M.R. if she returns home.

Meeting 2: Defining the ability to choose one's own residence

The first person to speak at this meeting is, once again, Brigitte. 'I've been thinking about what it means to say that someone is capable of deciding where she'll live, and I've concluded that it's essentially a negative matter. Ordinarily, people just decide where to live, and no one questions them. Beyond some really general factors that everyone must consider – like, can you afford it, and money's not an issue here – people may have thousands of different reasons for picking their residence. It's not like driving a car, where there are some things that every safe driver absolutely *must* be able to do. What we are really asking here is whether we are justified in challenging Ms M.R.'s *right* to decide where she'll live. So, here's my definition.' Brigitte then writes on the chalk-board in the meeting room:

> Incompetency to choose a place of residence is essentially the inability to appreciate the risk of harm to oneself, and others, that will arise from living in a particular place or circumstances.

'Now,' continues Brigitte, 'with Ms M.R. the real concerns all arise from her medical problems. But the competency we want to get at is different from competency to consent to treatment. We want to know whether she can apply information about her medical condition to the choice of her residence. So we need to know,' and she continues writing on the board:

1   Does she have the ability to appreciate the risks that she will face if she lives alone?

2   Can she recognize the range of residential alternatives open to her, for example, nursing home, seniors' apartment building, her own apartment?

3   Does she have reasons for her choice of residence?

Here, Brigitte pauses and adds, 'It's really up to her, you know. Maybe she wants to run risks for the sake of her independence.'

The others react immediately to this point. Harriet speaks for all of the others. 'This woman wants to live. She knows about nursing homes and seniors' apartments, but she says that she really loves her own apartment and wants her privacy. She thinks that she can look after herself. She's not choosing independence over safety – she's convinced that she can have both.'

'Fine, fine,' said Brigitte. 'That focuses us in on the real issue as far as choice of residence is concerned: Does she have the ability to assess the risks that she will run if she chooses to live alone?'

'But,' she continues, 'we should recognize that this assessment involves more than simple competence to choose a place of residence. We're also assessing her ability to thrive in the place where she chooses to live. And that raises separate concerns. Let's assume that she is at risk if she lives alone. We still have to know,' and here Brigitte again writes on the board:

1   Has she the ability to recognize risk and to accept help in coping with it?

2   Has she the ability to consider whether the assistance she requires to avoid harm is actually available to her?

The others agree that Brigitte's criteria are reasonable. On the basis of the information available to them they agree, subject to subsequent confirmation, that the real issues in the case are the ability to assess risk and to thrive in a chosen place of residence.

Having clarified the issues, the team then hears reports from Harriet and Jack.

Harriet begins with Ms M.R.'s knowledge of the risks to which she is exposed by living alone: 'It's clear to me, and to her nurses, that she knows what diabetes is and what might happen to her if she messes up on her diet or insulin. She says that she wants to go home and that she'll monitor her diet and drugs the way she did before her stroke.

The floor staff all think that her memory just isn't up to it.' Martin Smith interjects, 'Her doctors say the same thing. She wants both health and independence and the medical people say that if she really had the ability to understand her own condition she'd know that she can't have both.' 'I gave her my own MMS,' says Harriet (MMS is an acronym for a widely used screening test for cognitive deficiencies, the full name of which is the Mini-Mental Status Examination), 'and my results are the same as the test we already have. She has problems with memory and concentration, but she's not highly impaired – right on the borderline.'

Jack then speaks, 'Look, I agree with Brigitte's definitions but they're too abstract. And Ms M.R.'s ability to assess risk really overlaps with her ability to thrive. We need to focus more tightly on what she actually has to do for herself if she lives alone,' and he writes on the chalk board:

1   Purchase appropriate food and medications.

2   Eat the correct amount and kind of food at the correct time.

3   Take the correct amount of insulin at the correct time.

Jack resumes talking, 'She's got a niece who gives her a lot of help. Harriet got Ms M.R.'s permission for me to interview the niece – a nice woman. She's always bought Ms M.R.'s food and medicine for her, and she's going to keep doing it if her aunt goes home. I already spoke to the nutritionist at the hospital, and she's working out a diet plan and shopping list for the niece to use. So food is no problem. As for the insulin, Ms M.R.'s doctor telephones a prescription to a drug-store where the niece picks it up once a week and delivers it to her aunt. So, food and medicine are no problem.' He draws a line through point 1. 'She can get what she needs – the question is, can she use it?'

'Why not release her from hospital and see how she does?' asks Brigitte. Martin Smith replies (a little testily), 'Brigitte, you don't understand how sick this lady is. Her diabetes is really brittle – it wouldn't take much of a mistake to send her into a coma or shock. If we send her home she could be dead before we decide if she's competent.' Recovering his composure, he says, 'Look, I agree that the best possible test would be to send her home, but it's just not realistic. Whatever we do will have to be done in hospital.'

'I'm ahead of you,' says Jack. 'We can come pretty close to duplicating her home conditions here in the hospital. Let her niece buy her groceries and medicine just the way that she will if Ms M.R. goes home. We can keep the stuff in the Occupational Therapy department's test kitchen. She'll cook for herself and take her own medicine. The nurses can monitor her and prompt her if she fails badly enough to harm herself.'

The team agrees that this *task-specific test* would be an excellent approach. Harriet agrees to coordinate the experiment with the hospital staff, and Jack will make the appropriate arrangements with Mrs M.R.'s niece.

Meeting 3: Failure

One week later the team meets again. Harriet makes her report. 'This has been a miserable failure. The ward staff are furious with us – Ms M.R. is trying, but she is forgetful, and it makes a lot of work for them. They say we should have listened to them in the first place. She missed her insulin shots as often as she took them. She forgot to eat, or ate too much or not enough. A total, miserable, abject failure,' she concludes, unhappily.

'Well I'm not sure that you're right,' says Martin. 'The nurses tell me that if they give her instructions she follows them beautifully. She can execute well enough, she just can't remember what she's supposed to do. And this was only a one-week trial. Things did get a little better toward the end of the week. Ms M.R. may get better with practice. After all, people have been doing everything for her while she's been in the hospital.'

Brigitte asks, 'Is there any way of having someone give her instructions if she lives at home – you know, a home-care worker or someone like that?' Jack responds, 'You know, that's really a good idea. She does have her niece to remind her of things. And maybe she can follow written instructions just as well as she does the nurses' oral ones. The nutritionist already prepared a diet plan for her. Maybe we could prepare a total care plan – written instructions for diet and insulin – and see if she can follow it.' Brigitte objects, 'But doesn't this lady forget things? What makes you think she won't lose the list?'

'That's easy,' says Jack, 'we'll get the OT's to prepare a really huge list – big, big writing – that we can post on the door to her hospital room. At home we'll put it on her bedroom door and in her kitchen. *And* her niece can phone her first thing in the morning to remind her to check her list.' 'I think it's worth a try,' says Harriet, 'even though the ward staff are so peeved already that I'm going to have a hard time persuading them to go along with it.' The team agrees that Ms M.R. has not yet been given a fair chance and that the experiment should continue for another two weeks, using the list, so that Ms M.R. will have a significant opportunity to master her new routine.

The final meeting

After two weeks Harriet sends the following written report to each team member.

> The first three days of the test brought spotty results. Ms M.R. continued to forget to prepare her meals, or did so at the wrong time, and had to be prompted to take her medicine. But on the fourth day she got two meals and all her insulin injections right – with no prompting. By this time the staff were beginning to get enthusiastic, and were really encouraging her. By the fifth day she took perfectly good care of herself and continued to do so without a lapse for the rest of the two weeks. I can see no reason for any further meeting, unless others feel differently. While our test is not perfectly conclusive, there is now good reason to believe that Ms M.R. is right – with appropriate memory aids she can function independently. I vote that we file a report saying that she is competent so long as she uses the memory devices that Jack prepared.

To this report Martin Smith appends the following note:

> I agree with Harriet, although I am still a little worried about how she will do without people around to encourage and congratulate her. For this reason, I would like to recommend that Ms M.R. have a nurse to help her establish a routine during her first week at home and to stop by weekly thereafter to monitor her. Ms M.R. quite welcomes this assistance. I also think that the report should say that our conclusion is premised on her niece's willingness to continue helping with shopping.

The other members of the team agree with the conclusion stated in the report. Brigitte dissents on the recommendation about home nursing care, for which she thinks there is no demonstrated need. The report is filed in the terms that Harriet Campbell and Martin Smith have proposed. Ms M.R. returns to her own home.

Ms C.S.: Assessing competency to make health-care decisions

Ms C.S. (the woman who has multiple sclerosis and needs a feeding tube) has lost most of her physical abilities, but all those who care for her believe that she is mentally alert. She can neither speak nor write, and she will soon die unless she receives a feeding tube through which she can receive nutrition despite her inability to chew and swallow. Her death is imminent in any event, and a feeding tube involves a certain amount of discomfort. Unfortunately, no one discussed the possibility of a feeding tube with Ms C.S. while she was able to communicate her wishes, and so no one knows what her wishes are. Her physician is determined to give Ms C.S. the opportunity to make her own choice regarding the insertion of the tube and refers Ms C.S. for an assessment of her competency to make a health-care decision, hoping that the psychiatrist will find some way of establishing meaningful communication with her.

The hospital in which Ms C.S. lives does not have the money to purchase sophisticated speech aids. Its one speech therapist works only part-time and is unavailable to help the psychiatrist with his assessment. He has however reviewed her notes and case reports on Ms C.S. and will also confirm his findings with her. But in the circumstances he cannot delay the assessment long enough to permit her to assist him. And he does find a way to communicate with Ms C.S. She is able to use her left hand and arm; with some difficulty she is able to point to the word yes or no, each of which is painted in large block letters on a sign that is placed close to her in bed. With this simple device she can respond to questions.

Competency to make a health-care decision

There are two essential elements of competency to consent to health care:

1   Is the person able to understand the information that is relevant to making a decision about treatment?
2   Is the person able to appreciate the likely consequences of accepting or refusing treatment?

In sum, a person who is competent to consent to medical treatment must have the ability to understand information and to apply it to his or her personal situation. The above formulation is based substantially on the province of Ontario's new Consent to Treatment Act and has been selected because it is compatible with the general approach of this book to competency assessment. The test reflects current legal approaches to capacity assessment because it focuses on the *ability* to comprehend information and appreciate consequences, as opposed to *actual* comprehension and appreciation. But many statutory and judicial tests for competency to consent to treatment differ from this one, and competency assessors must seek advice from a qualified person on the standard that they should apply in their locality. For example, some statutes require people actually to understand relevant information and potential consequences. Others require competent people only to understand the 'nature' of their illness. In practice, however, there is often considerable overlap between different legal standards. So, for example, an ill person who cannot acknowledge in general terms that he or she is ill could neither be said to appreciate the nature of his or her illness nor to have the ability to appreciate the likely consequences of accepting or rejecting treatment.

The presumption in favor of life

Lawyers and ethicists often apply the presumption in favor of life to cases like that of Ms C.S. The following assessment of Ms C.S. ignores the presumption, but it is important to understand what that presumption is and the reasons for omitting it from the assessment of Ms C.S.

The presumption may be thought of as a rule that directs health-care providers to favor the preservation of life in the absence of a cogent reason for acting otherwise. A corollary of the rule is that it is reasonable to assume that rational people making their own health-care decisions will generally choose to preserve their own lives. The presumption in favor of life is thus sometimes relied on to justify the administration of life-saving care without any substitute consent to an incapable person whose own wishes regarding the care are unknown. A classic example is the provision of emergency care to a person who is unconscious following an automobile accident. The presumption is also sometimes applied in assessing competency to consent to life-sustaining treatment. In this context the presumption is used to justify the application of a lower standard of mental competency to a person who accepts life-sustaining care than is applied to a person who rejects it. The reason for doing so is the assumption that competent people will generally decide in favor of preserving their life. In effect, the lawyers and ethicists who apply the presumption in this way view competency not merely as task-specific but also as decision-specific.

The psychiatrist decides to treat Ms C.S.'s case as though there were no presumption in favor of life, in part so that he can avoid becoming embroiled in the vexed debate over the ethics of end-of-life care. But there are more important reasons for leaving the presumption aside in this case. First, in practice people are often too quick to assume that they cannot, or need not, elicit the wishes and assess the competency of people who have difficulty communicating. Ms C.S.'s physician knows that he can rely on the presumption if need be, that is, if he cannot establish reliable communication with her or if she proves to be incompetent to make her own decisions; but before he does so he feels ethically bound not merely to assess her competency but also to try to establish her own wishes. The assessment of Ms C.S. thus serves two purposes. It is an attempt to permit Ms C.S. to make her own decision as well as an assessment of her competency to do so.

For the purposes of this book, moreover, Mrs F.C.'s case is meant to be a model for assessing people who have difficulty communicating. Many such cases do not involve life-sustaining care, and so they cannot be resolved by applying the presumption in favor of life. Nonetheless, people should not be surprised to find the presumption in favor of life applied in actual cases. No conclusions about its validity or its proper application should be drawn from the following case.

The assessment

In addition to assessing Ms C.S.'s ability to assimilate and apply information, the psychiatrist must assess the *reliability* of the communication that is established with her and the adequacy of the questions asked. Reliable communication has been established with Ms C.S. if she is able to say what she means. The questions asked of her are adequate if they present her with the option that *she* most wants. An assessor of someone like Ms C.S. proceeds by putting a series of alternatives to her. For example, she might be asked whether she wants a feeding tube now. If her answer is no, she would then be asked whether she wishes to have a feeding tube at some later time. If she answers yes to this question she would be asked whether she would like to have it sooner than one month from now. The risk of such a process is that the option that Ms C.S. really wants may never be offered to her. To safeguard against this risk Ms C.S. is continually asked whether the choice that she most wants has yet been included among those offered to her.

The assessor realizes that the most difficult element of competency to establish will be the ability of Ms C.S. to make medical decisions based on her own preferences, that is, her ability to make choices. The difficulty lies in the fact that this ability is best assessed by asking a person to explain the reasons for the decision that he or she proposes to make, and Ms C.S. cannot easily communicate her reasoning. The assessor overcomes this problem by assessing Ms C.S. on two separate occasions. On each occasion she gave him the same answers. He took the persistence of her wishes as evidence that she had reasons for her decision – that her decision was based on her own persistent beliefs and opinions – even though she was unable to communicate them to him. In legal terms, the physician correctly assumed that the burden of proving incompetency fell on him, and he relied on the presumption of competency when he could find no evidence of incompetency.

The physician began his assessment by testing the reliability of the communication he had established with Ms C.S. He did this by asking her several questions to which he already knew the answers. For example, Ms C.S. is fifty-eight years old, but the physician asked her whether she is sixty-four years old; she answered no, thus confirming that her pointing was indeed meaningful communication. After several such satisfactory answers, he asked her a series of questions about feeding tubes, to ascertain that she had all the information she needed to make her decision. He asked her many questions about the potential risks and benefits of the insertion of a feeding tube: for example, whether a feeding tube would help her gain weight; whether the feeding tube would cause her to lose weight; whether she wanted to gain weight, etc. It became clear that Ms C.S. understood the potential benefits and discomforts of a feeding tube; as well, she consistently indicated that she wanted the feeding tube inserted. Satisfied that Ms C.S. possessed adequate information, the psychiatrist then explored her ability to consent (or refuse consent) to the insertion of one. To start, he asked Ms C.S. whether her physician had told her about feeding tubes and asked whether she wanted to have one inserted; she answered yes to both questions. On the first day he probed her answer gently, seeking her response to statements like: a feeding tube will prolong my life; a feeding tube will not prolong my life; I wish to prolong my life, etc. On the second day the psychiatrist took a more aggressive approach. He told Ms C.S. that her physician wanted to perform surgery on her left hand. He knew she has much better control of her left hand than of her right, and asked whether she wanted this surgery. Ms C.S. responded no, and her facial expression conveyed dismay and confusion at such a suggestion; the psychiatrist immediately told her that her physician really did not advise such an operation, and he explained why he had asked this misleading, and upsetting, question. On the basis of her reply to this one question the psychiatrist now knew that she has the abilities to distinguish a feeding tube from other kinds of treatment (because she wants a feeding tube but not an operation on her hand), to distinguish treatment that is appropriate to her condition from treatment that is not (she knew that there was nothing wrong with her left hand and refused the operation but also knew that she could not swallow or chew and consented to the insertion of a feeding tube), and to resist treatment that her physician recommends but that she believes is inappropriate. Ms C.S., concluded the psychiatrist, has the ability to assimilate medical information, to apply it to the circumstances of her own life, and to make independent decisions about her treatment. The physician decided that Ms C.S. is competent to consent to the insertion of a feeding tube, and that she consents to the procedure.

Common errors in competency assessment

So far, we have discussed the methods and principles that ought to be applied to a formal competency assessment. But competency assessments are not always properly conducted. This chapter concludes with a checklist that may help assessors provide good assessments. It can also be used by other people to judge the quality of the assessment that they, or a relative or friend, have received.

1 Authority Does the person conducting a formal competency assessment have the training to do so? Does the assessor have the legal authority to provide any follow-up reports that may be required for legal purposes (for example, to support a guardianship application)?

2 Informing the patient Has the patient been told that he or she is to be assessed? Has he or she consented to the assessment?

3 Purpose Does the proposed competency assessment serve an immoral or illegal purpose?

4 Necessity Is the proposed assessment necessary? That is, is there reason to believe that the person is at risk of harm? Is there reason to believe that, if found incompetent, he or she will have access to care that would not otherwise be available?

5 Testing Is the assessor relying solely on psychological tests that are not task-specific to determine whether a person lacks a particular competency? For example, is the assessor relying on a test like the MSE to see whether a person is financially incompetent?

6 Task-specificity Is the assessor using tests of task-specific competency that are not trivial? Do they replicate as closely as possible the actual circumstances in which the person performs the tested task?

7 Informal support In designing tests of task-specific competence, is the assessor taking into consideration the informal support the person being assessed may receive from willing relatives and friends?

8 False inferences Is the assessor concluding that a person is incompetent only because the person has a disease or illness that generally does render people incompetent? Have tests been made to determine the abilities of this one individual who is being assessed?

9 Focus on abilities Is the assessor concluding that a person is incompetent only because psychological testing shows that the person has lost mental abilities without which people usually are incompetent? Has the assessor conducted task-specific tests of these abilities?

10 One-shot assessments Is the assessor allowing adequate time for a thorough investigation? One-shot assessments are generally inadequate except in cases where the assessed person is either manifestly capable or manifestly incapable.

11 Assessor-produced incompetency Is the assessor doing something that prevents the person from displaying his or her true abilities? In this connection, several questions may be asked.

    i Is the person comfortable with the assessor? For example, is a woman who is uncomfortable discussing her private affairs with a man being assessed by a man?

    ii Is the assessor allowing for nervousness in the person who is being assessed?

    iii Is the assessment being conducted while a person is temporarily incompetent? Is the person still suffering from the results of a recent accident or medical emergency, or taking a medication that impairs his or her thinking?

    iv Is the assessor accommodating the person's physical frailty, or are sessions going on so long that the person becomes fatigued and unable to perform at his or her best?

    v Is the assessor confusing fluctuating competency and total incompetency (a special risk when dealing with elderly people)? Does a particular task require the person to be continuously competent, or is it sufficient for the person to be competent only while issuing an instruction that others will follow?

12 Seeking the best possible performance Is the assessor taking all reasonable steps to allow the person to perform at his or her best? Again, several questions may be asked.

    i Has the assessment been scheduled for a time when the person is generally at his or her best?

    ii Is the person being encouraged to take advantage of aids that he or she ordinarily relies on to overcome disabilities? That is, did the assessor ask how the person has managed to perform tasks in the past despite suffering from mental disabilities?

    iii Is the assessor prepared to schedule a home interview for a person who becomes disoriented outside his or her own home? This question is particularly apt when an elderly person has been assessed; older people are often much more comfortable at home and so perform better there.

    iv Is the assessor giving the person appropriate help? For example, is a person with memory problems being provided with reasonable prompting or appropriate memory aids?

13 Meeting the case against them Is the person properly informed of the assessor's results and conclusions and given fair opportunity to rebut them?

14 Correct reasoning vs. correct answers Does the assessor have a good grasp of the person's reasoning? Is the assessor inferring that a seemingly wrong answer proves that the person is incapable, without considering, (a) that the person may have his or her own perfectly good reasons, which the assessor has failed to appreciate, for the answer; or (b) that the person may simply need some advice or information; or (c) that the problem may lie in the test being applied or in the manner of its application?

15 Choices not correctness Is the assessor treating his own disapproval of a person's choices as proof that the person is incompetent?

CHAPTER SIX

Guardianship and other imposed care

When people who have not planned for their own care while competent become chronically incompetent, it is sometimes necessary to have a judge appoint a guardian for them. In doing so, the judge will often rely on reports from a competency assessor. People who seek assessments that may lead to guardianship, and the assessors who perform them, should therefore be especially conscious of their duty to safeguard individual liberty. To understand why this is so, it is necessary to consider the nature of guardianship, and especially the loss of individual rights that it entails. As a general rule, one should satisfy oneself that there is no reasonable alternative form of care available before considering guardianship.

There are in fact other forms of non-consensual care that may be considered when dealing with an incompetent person, some of which are discussed in general terms later. Nevertheless, this chapter focuses on guardianship. This is so, first, because some form of guardianship is universally available in North America and so too is the problem of deciding whether and when to impose it. There are also secondary, but still weighty, reasons for emphasizing guardianship. Principal among these is demographics. The North American population is getting increasingly older overall, and the incidence of dementia increases dramatically with age. Those who care for a demented person often require the ongoing authority to make substitute decisions on that person's behalf. In many cases guardianship is the best, and in some cases it is the only, means of obtaining such authority. In any event, the same concerns that arise with guardianship are also often relevant to other forms of non-consensual intervention and decision making.

Guardianship

The details of guardianship legislation differ markedly from province to province and state to state, but the purpose of guardianship does not. A guardian (who may also be called, according to local law and practice, a curator, committee, conservator, or fiduciary) is a person to whom a judge grants the power of making decisions regarding the finances or property, or personal care, or both, of a person who is incapable of making his or her own decisions. Guardians are generally under a legal duty to safeguard the interests and well-being of the incompetent person for whom they make decisions. In short, guardianship is a legal mechanism by which a competent person may obtain the legal authority to make decisions for an incompetent person.

Incompetency and incapacity

Guardianship laws typically define the nature or degree of incompetency that justifies depriving individuals of the right to make their own decisions and appointing a guardian for them. Most laws refer to a person who requires a guardian as either 'mentally incompetent' or 'mentally incapacitated,' but the definitions of these terms have evolved over time. Older statutes tend to relate incapacity to particular diagnoses or illnesses, and so they define an incompetent as a person who, because of mental illness, mental retardation, senility, excessive use of drugs or alcohol, or other physical or mental incapacity, is incapable of either managing his property or caring for himself or both. More modern legislation recognizes that a diagnosis is alone no proof of incompetency, and so incompetency is defined in relation to the ability to perform tasks. Thus, some legislation defines a mentally incapacitated person as someone whose ability to receive and evaluate information effectively or to make and to communicate decisions is impaired to such an extent that he or she (1) lacks the capacity to meet essential requirements for his or her physical health or safety; and (2) is unable to manage his or her financial resources. Still more recent laws not only define incompetency in terms of the inability to perform tasks but provide for the possibility of partial incompetency. They do not treat personal care as a single, monolithic entity but break it down into subsidiary components such as nutrition, shelter, and medical care. In contrast, older laws recognize only two broad categories of incapacity – financial and personal care. Thus, the most recent laws may define a mentally incapacitated person as someone whose ability to receive and evaluate information effectively or to communicate decisions is impaired to such an extent that he or she lacks the capacity to manage all or some of his or her financial resources or to meet all or some essential requirements for his or her physical health, safety, habilitation, or therapeutic needs without court-ordered assistance or the appointment of a guardian. Some recent laws provide helpful guidance to judges and assessors by specifying that age, eccentricity, poverty, or medical diagnosis alone are insufficient reasons for the appointment of a guardian. Guardianship law increasingly defines incompetency in a way that is consistent with the principles on which this book is based.

Guardianship legislation increasingly tends to recognize that competency must be assessed in relation to particular tasks and in relation to the circumstances of the particular individuals' own lives. Many older statutes, however, incorporate vague or misleading definitions of incompetency. In applying older statutes both assessors, and the relatives and friends of incompetent people, must supply the appropriate principles and standards that the law itself does not explicitly incorporate. But even a law that explicitly incorporates clear and justifiable definitions of incompetency will be effective only when its *general* directions as well as the specifics are followed in the assessments that lead up to guardianship applications. Even more important, the mere fact that the legal requirements for the appointment of a guardian may be satisfied does not always mean that a guardianship application is justified. This is particularly true in relation to the older and vaguer type of guardianship legislation, but it may also apply to more recent legislation. For example, a person may be incompetent or incapacitated according to a legal definition, but quite willing to accept the assistance needed to protect himself or herself from harm. Without some compelling reason to justify a guardianship application, the principle of the least-restrictive alternative dictates that no guardianship application should be brought on behalf such a person.

As a general rule, people who are considering seeking the guardianship of another person should first undertake their own informal competency assessment based on the principles outlined in chapter 4. The purpose of this assessment is to consider whether a guardianship application is both necessary and justified. As well, it is particularly important for assessors who perform formal competency assessments that may lead to a guardianship order to consider and follow the principles and practices outlined in chapter 5.

Guardianship and liberty

In general, the more recent guardianship statutes define incompetency (often called incapacity) as actual functional incapacity – namely, a person's inability to make decisions in the circumstances of his or her own life. These laws often also incorporate the notion of task-specific incompetency, that is, they recognize that a person may be incompetent in respect of some tasks, but competent in respect of others. In contrast, older laws tend to view incompetency as a global, all-or-nothing condition. Some laws offer more explicit and comprehensible guidance to the judges and competency assessors who apply them than others do. In applying older guardianship laws an especially heavy onus falls on the shoulders of applicants for guardianship, and on competency assessors, to ensure that liberty is not unduly restricted. But a heavy onus also falls on the shoulders of those who apply more modern and justifiable guardianship laws. Even with statutes that incorporate sound definitions of incompetency or incapacity, guardianship may result in the unnecessary deprivation of individual liberty.

Rescinding guardianship

Although virtually all guardianship laws provide that a judge may rescind a guardianship order if a person no longer requires a guardian, in practice once a guardianship order has been made it tends to remain in effect. It is not entirely clear why this is so. Perhaps guardianship is sought only for very deteriorated people, or, alternatively, perhaps those found to be mentally incompetent are not given sufficient opportunity to challenge their guardians' authority. In any case, those who seek to impose guardianship on another, or who perform assessments leading up to guardianship applications, should consider that once initiated guardianship is likely to be permanent.

Guardianship and assessment

A guardian is appointed after it has been proved to a judge that a person is legally incompetent or incapacitated. Often, some of this 'proof' will be provided in the form of oral or written statements from

the person's relatives or friends. The laws generally require that incapacity must also be established by way of an oral or written report from
a health-care professional who has assessed the allegedly incompetent
person. Older laws may require that these assessments be performed
by a physician, or more specifically by a psychiatrist, but newer laws
tend to expand the classes of assessors to include psychologists and
other non-physician health-care professionals. Some statutes allow a
judge to appoint an individual (variously referred to as a visitor, an
investigator, or a guardian *ad litem*) to undertake what amounts to a
functional assessment of an allegedly incompetent person; these laws
may permit a judge to rely on a social worker or similar professional
for the assessment.

Regardless of their professional affiliations, all assessors must be
conscious of the implications of the assessments that they perform.
Even under modern guardianship statutes it may be difficult for judges
to look very far beyond the assessment reports that they receive. If
competency assessments are thorough, fair, and comprehensive, it is
likely that judicial decisions about the appointment of guardians will
be sound. But the converse is also true; if the assessments that a judge
receives are hasty, unfair, and superficial, it is likely that judicial decisions about the appointments of guardians will be unsound.

Safeguards in guardianship law

In addition to defining incompetency more precisely and justifiably
than older laws did, modern legislation also safeguards the liberty of
allegedly incompetent people in other ways. Modern laws often explicitly grant procedural rights to allegedly incompetent people that
older laws do not. They may ensure, for example, the right to receive
notice of a proposed guardianship hearing, the right to be present at
the hearing, or the right to be represented by counsel who will follow
the client's instructions rather than act in what the counsel believes to
be the client's 'best interests.' As already mentioned, some legislation
even permits the judge to commission a functional competency assessment of the kind advocated by this book. Some states have established
public agencies that discharge this function. As well, modern legislation tends to require or permit guardians' powers to be limited so that
they are proportional with an incapacitated person's disabilities. They
may separate guardianship of property and finances from guardianship
of the person, so that one may be instituted without the other. They

may also separate the various aspects of personal guardianship – nutrition, medical treatment, residence, etc. – and provide for a guardian to make decisions only in respect to one or some combination of these matters. This kind of guardianship is often called limited or partial guardianship, and under such laws a guardian of the person might, for example, have the power to make decisions about residence but not about medical care.

Modern laws may also incorporate various mechanisms to ensure that guardians use their powers honestly and carefully. The guardians may be prohibited from consenting to various procedures, for example, or they may be required to file accounts, care plans, or notices of change of residence, as, for example, when a person is moved from his or her own apartment to a nursing home. To summarize, older forms of guardianship are an all-or-nothing proposition, but more modern ones provide for what amounts to task-specific guardianship that corresponds to task-specific incompetencies of particular individuals. Modern guardianship legislation takes the protection of individual liberty, and the provision of the least-restrictive alternative form of care, more seriously than its predecessors did.

This does not, however, lessen the burden imposed on competency assessors. Indeed, these modern laws actually demand more of assessors because they call for assessments to be proper, task-specific, and functional. One must, however, recognize that guardianship laws are not self-executing, and it is wrong to assume that the law in practice accurately reflects the law that is on the books. Bad guardianship laws may, in the hands of well-educated and thoughtful judges, assessors, and guardians, produce good results; but good laws, if applied by judges, assessors, and guardians who do not understand what competency is, and who are unfamiliar with proper assessment methods, may produce bad results. Proper judicial decisions in guardianship cases depend on good competency assessments.

Moreover, practical considerations may reduce or eliminate the effectiveness of recent innovations in guardianship laws. Some critics complain, for example, that judges do not very often use the power to make limited guardianship orders, and they suggest or imply that this is caused by judicial ignorance or judicial unwillingness to adapt to modern approaches to incompetency. It is reasonable to think that these complaints are overstated. It may be that many people delay seeking a guardianship order until the incompetent person is very deteriorated, thus making an order for complete guardianship the only reasonable alternative open to the judge who decides the case. Even when a person is not completely incompetent, when the order is made there may be sound practical reasons why his or her friends or relatives might seek, and a judge might grant, an order for complete guardianship. It is expensive to bring an application for guardianship, and it may be ruinously so to bring repeated applications to expand a guardian's powers as a person's incompetence progresses. As well, judges may fear that if those who bring guardianship applications are forced to pay too high a price for their willingness to aid incompetent people, they simply will not bring the applications and may abandon their relatives or attempt to pass responsibility for their relatives' care over to public agencies or institutions. Moreover, the already hard-pressed North American judicial system can ill afford a scheme for guardianship appointments that may require multiple applications, and so consume much valuable court time. As a result, in fairness to relatives and friends, out of a practical judgment that rigorously applied laws may deter would-be caregivers, and to preserve the efficient functioning of the courts, judges may be reluctant to make limited guardianship orders.

The current willingness to experiment with measures to improve the quality of guardianship orders, and of guardianship itself, are entirely praiseworthy. But it is both reasonable and prudent to be skeptical about how effective these new laws and innovations will be. Careful assessors of competency, indeed thoughtful people generally, will assume that guardianship involves a significant loss of legal rights and that it will (in common with all forms of substitute decision making) involve some risk of abuse, including the possibility that the guardianship will not be rescinded even if the incompetent person recovers competency. People, and particularly assessors, should think of guardianship as a measure of last resort for the care of an incompetent person.

Alternatives to guardianship

Adult protection statutes

Adult protection legislation is becoming increasingly prevalent as the population ages and the need to establish public measures to help abused or neglected elderly people receives more public recognition.

Such legislation has several common features. Typically these laws establish a public agency or institution to investigate allegations that an adult is being abused or neglected or impose this duty on some existing agency or institution. In these laws abuse or neglect are often defined in fairly broad terms that encompass a range of financial, physical, and emotional harms. Some, but not all, laws permit public intervention in an abused or neglected person's life only if the person is incompetent to protect himself or herself.

If an investigation establishes that a person is in fact suffering from abuse or neglect the laws establish a range of increasingly intrusive remedies that may be applied. The range begins with a mere offer of assistance that a person may either accept or reject, through various measures for short-term non-consensual emergency intervention (for example, removing an abusive person from the place where the victim resides), to measures for long-term non-consensual intervention that are comparable to court-appointed guardianship. Some laws permit a public agency or official to apply to become a person's guardian.

Adult protection statutes thus may extend to matters that fall outside the scope of this book (for example, spouse abuse), but they also provide a means of obtaining help for incompetent people. Indeed one of the principal goals of such legislation everywhere is to provide for incompetent elderly people. For the purposes of this book it is helpful to think of adult protection laws as akin to a publicly initiated, funded, and overseen form of guardianship. The proper application of adult protection statutes to incompetent people will often be as dependent on thorough, fair, complete competency assessment as the imposition of guardianship is. In fact, some laws explicitly make incompetency a ground for intervention. Even where the laws do not impose such a condition it will sometimes be helpful to assess informally the competency of someone who seems to be neglected before making a report to an adult protection agency; sometimes a person who appears to be neglected is simply living an eccentric life. And even when a person is beyond doubt abused or neglected, a formal or informal assessment of competency will often be essential to establish the range of decisions that the person is capable of making, and from that the range of necessary and justified state intervention in his or her life. In other words, an informal or formal assessment is necessary to match the kind and extent of assistance offered to the person's needs. Although the following discussion does not explicitly mention the application of adult protection laws, much of it is directly relevant to those who must decide whether to initiate investigations under such laws, and also to public officials who provide assistance to abused or neglected people. The discussion of informal assessment in chapter 4 is similarly relevant.

Civil commitment

'Civil commitment' as used here, refers to the legal process by which a person is confined without his or her consent, and perhaps against his or her will, for care and treatment in a psychiatric hospital or some comparable facility. Many incompetent people do not fit the common statutory criteria for involuntary hospitalization, and there are many reasons why civil commitment is often the wrong response to the needs of incompetent people. Civil commitment is mentioned here only to identify it as a measure that may sometimes have to be used to care for elderly incompetent people but that should be viewed as a last resort.

In the past civil commitment was sometimes used to obtain shelter and care for older people who were too ill or frail to protect themselves. Even now civil commitment is, unfortunately, sometimes the only way to protect elderly demented people who have no relatives and friends to assist them. But even where such people may legally be committed, the appropriate institutions and facilities for their care may not be available. Civil commitment laws and psychiatric facilities are increasingly designed to provide crisis care, not long-term, ongoing care of the kind required by people who suffer from chronic mental illnesses or disabilities. As well, civil commitment laws often do not apply to elderly incompetent people who need, but refuse, care. As a broad generalization, admittedly subject to many qualifications and exceptions, it is reasonable to say that civil commitment is of limited applicability to incompetent people aside from those suffering from major psychiatric illnesses like schizophrenia or manic depression, and it is often of little use even with these people. Civil commitment should generally be considered only as a short-term solution to the problems of incompetent people, a wholly inadequate substitute for a properly thought out and executed plan of *long-term* care.

When to consider guardianship

People should consider imposing guardianship on others only when it is truly necessary to do so. In general, guardianship should be considered only for people:

1a Whose mental incompetence has deprived them of the ability to react appropriately to the circumstances and situations that commonly arise in their daily affairs, or who may reasonably be expected to do so, and who are therefore exposed, or are exposing others to, an intolerable risk of harm. Harm, in this context, means unpleasant or hurtful consequences that the allegedly incompetent person would ordinarily strive to avoid and that reasonable people would likely object to having another impose on them without their consent.

  b Who do not recognize the risks that they are running themselves or imposing on others, or who will not accept measures to reduce or eliminate them.

  c Who have not appointed a substitute decision maker who has adequate powers to address the problem, and who are at the time incapable of, or unwilling to, consider making such an appointment.

2 Who are incompetent, who require the service of a guardian, and who while competent to do so expressed a desire to have one appointed for them if necessary.

3 Who have expressed wishes regarding the care that they should receive in the event of their incompetency, who are now incompetent, and whose decisions can be executed only if a guardian is appointed for them. For example, a person might have expressed a desire to have a friend make decisions for him in the event of incompetency, yet local laws will automatically give the right to make decisions to someone else unless the chosen decider seeks a guardianship order.

In brief, guardianship should ordinarily be considered only for people who are both incompetent and at risk of harm to themselves or others, or when its imposition is in accordance with a person's competent wishes.

When properly applied, guardianship should not deprive individuals of their independence but merely recognize that they have already lost it to mental incompetency. It is, of course, one thing to state a general formula like this one and another to apply it in reality. The range of circumstances in which a guardianship order may justifiably be sought is enormous. There are, however, three common situations where guardianship is often both necessary and justified.

1   For a person who is incapable of making an urgent decision, who has not previously appointed a substitute decision maker, and who is now incompetent or unwilling to appoint one. For example, it would be appropriate to appoint a financial guardian for a person who is incapable of paying his taxes and will face a ruinous penalty if no one else does it for him.

2   For a person who is placing himself or herself or others at intolerable risk of physical injury and who will not accept measures that will reduce the risk to tolerable levels. It would be appropriate, for example, to appoint a personal guardian, with the power to determine the place or circumstances of residence, for a person who has set three fires in his kitchen while frying food, and who refuses to consider alternative cooking methods.

3   For a person who is now, or will likely soon be, extremely or completely incompetent, as may be the case with people in the final stages of Alzheimer's disease – that is, for people who are manifestly incapable of making almost any decision, or who will soon be in this condition.

To repeat: guardianship is an extreme measure that should be imposed only if there are weighty reasons for doing so.

The decision to impose guardianship should take account of more than simply the risk of harm. The risk of harm that an individual is exposed to without a guardian must be weighed against the risk to individual liberty that guardianship may entail. In other words, when making the decision about whether or not to seek a guardianship order, it is important to make the attempt to put risk in a proper perspective. More precisely, one must ask whether a particular risk or threat of harm really is serious enough to justify stripping a person of some (and perhaps many) ordinary rights. There is no easy or automatic test by which this judgment may be made. However, if the reasons for considering guardianship are clear, and some common errors can be avoided, the ultimate decision is much more likely to be fair and justifiable.

Risk

The decision whether or not a person needs a guardian often involves risk assessment, and it should follow the principles discussed in chapters 4 and 5. Two of the common errors discussed in earlier chapters are worth reconsidering in this connection. These are:

1 Exaggerating the risk that a person, for whose well-being the assessor considers himself or herself to be responsible, is actually exposed to.

This is particularly common when the person has already suffered some real (albeit often not serious) harm. Too often, others then tend to become irrationally closed to the possibility that the person is mentally competent and has reasons for exposing himself or herself to risk.

2 Assuming that guardianship is the only, or the most reasonable, way of reducing intolerable risk to a tolerable level.

People tend to seek the safest possible form of care for others who are at risk of harm, rather than the form of care that combines an acceptable level of safety with the least restriction of liberty. Assessors should be especially critical of the reasoning by which they may conclude that a person is at grave risk that can be eliminated only by the appointment of a guardian. Assessors should also be aware of the legal alternatives to guardianship (such as the execution of a durable power of attorney). They should consider whether a person who might otherwise require a guardian is willing and competent to make some arrangement for his or her care and protection.

Risk assessment is an art that requires the exercise of judgment. And just as it is possible to exaggerate risk, it is also possible to understate it. As much as it is important to be slow to conclude that another is at unacceptable risk of harm, it is vital not to be dogmatic in ignoring or underestimating the gravity of a condition or problem. A common area of concern is extreme memory loss, and there is often good reason to worry about the safety of a person who suffers from this disability. When their dementia is very advanced, or if they have a severe brain injury, the memories of some people are so impaired that they cannot remember their own acts long enough to appreciate their consequences. Some demented people have such bad memories that they forget that they have lit a cigarette by the time the match flares out. But even people whose memory loss is less extreme may pose a real danger to themselves and others. A person with extreme memory loss may forget, for example, having turned on a stove burner and will leave it burning. Compounding the danger, people with severe memory loss often deny that they have acted dangerously because they cannot recognize the dangerous behavior as their own: someone who cannot remember having turned on a stove burner cannot be expected to acknowledge neglecting to turn it off. People with extreme memory loss thus often cannot recognize the risks to which they expose themselves and others, and so can see no reason why they need or should accept help. Some of them will be safe only if they live in controlled circumstances where they have no access to appliances or implements that they are likely to misuse. Guardianship is often the only realistic form of care for people whose memory loss has effectively deprived them of self-control.

To sum up, in determining whether some form of involuntary care is justified for an individual, it is necessary to assess the risk of harm to which he or she is exposed without a guardian and to balance that risk against the threat that involuntary care poses to liberty. When performing such assessments people must guard themselves against any temptation they may feel to exaggerate risk, and they should consider alternative forms of care that may be effective but less restrictive of liberty than guardianship will be.

An example of guardianship

Mr L.H.: Civil commitment and guardianship

The following case illustrates the application of civil commitment and guardianship laws (in this case, those of the province of Ontario) to resolve a crisis. The primary purpose of this case is to illustrate the difficulties that may arise when people fail to make timely plans, well in advance of need, for the care of an incompetent person and to encourage people to plan for their own care and protection in the event of incompetency.

Mr L.H. is the elderly widower who lives with his daughter (D.) and son-in-law (S.). He has a progressive dementia, and he is quite disoriented and forgetful. For some time he has, without justification, accused D. and S. of stealing from him. His accusations are becoming more persistent, and he frequently suffers from panic attacks. As well he has recently begun to wander. Two days ago he left his daughter's house at 3 a.m.; it was very cold outside, and he was wearing only pajamas and slippers. D. and S. called the police when they discovered his absence. Mr L.H. was found at 9 a.m. wandering miles from home; he was taken to the hospital, treated for the effects of exposure, and released. D. and S. had decided before this incident that Mr L.H. should live in a nursing home, and they had even located an appropriate one that would soon have a bed for him. They had arranged to have Mr L.H.'s competency assessed for the purpose of bringing a guardianship application, but the assessment has not yet been conducted. There is no time to perform such an assessment now, for if Mr L.H. is not moved to a secure institution he may again wander from home, but might not be found before he freezes to death. However, Mr L.H. refuses to move voluntarily to a nursing home, and so he cannot be placed in one until D. and S. become his guardians. In desperation S. calls the family's physician for advice.

Involuntary psychiatric hospitalization

The physician (Dr A.) tells S. that Mr L.H. can probably be admitted into a psychiatric hospital as an involuntary patient and held there until D. and S. become his guardians and place him in a nursing home. Mr L.H. lives in Ontario, and Ontario's Mental Health Act allows a physician to apply for the psychiatric assessment of a person whom the physician has reasonable and probable grounds to believe has (among other possibilities) shown a lack of competence to care for himself or herself, and whom in the physician's opinion is suffering from a 'mental disorder of a nature or quality that will likely result in ... serious bodily harm to the person.' Mr L.H. suffers from dementia, which is a mental disorder. His behavior is caused by his dementia, and it has already placed him at risk of serious bodily harm and is likely to do so again. Still, Dr A. must examine Mr L.H. himself (he has not seen him for several months) to confirm that Mr L.H. really is as demented as S. says he is. At the examination Mr L.H. is extremely demented, so Dr A. arranges for his admission to a psychiatric hospital and completes the form that will allow the hospital to hold him for an involuntary psychiatric assessment. At the hospital Mr L.H. is again assessed by a psychiatrist (Dr B.) who shares Dr A.'s conclusions. Mr L.H. refuses to remain in the hospital, so Dr B. completes a form that allows him to be held as an involuntary patient. Mr L.H. has now been civilly committed.

The physicians and Mr L.H.'s children agree that the hospital is just a stop-gap measure until a guardianship order is obtained and Mr L.H. is moved to a nursing home.

Financial certification

Having admitted Mr L.H. to the psychiatric hospital as an involuntary patient, Dr B. now has a legal obligation to assess his financial competency. Mr L.H.'s memory and judgment are so severely impaired that he is clearly financially incompetent. Dr B. files a certificate of financial incompetence with the public trustee, the public official who has the duty to manage the finances and property of (among others) psychiatric patients who have been certified as incompetent. An official from the public trustee's office contacts Mrs L.H. and they arrange a meeting. The bulk of Mr L.H.'s assets are in Canada Savings Bonds and term deposit certificates. Ready cash is held in a joint account, of which Mr L.H. and his daughter are the signatories. D. deposits Mr L.H.'s pension and social security checks into this account and pays for his necessities from it. D. supplies all Mr L.H.'s financial records to the official, including a list of his assets and the deposit book for the joint savings account. She reviews all this material with the official and explains that she wishes to become Mr L.H.'s guardian. The officer is mildly critical of her inability to produce receipts to show how she has spent her father's money, but is otherwise satisfied with the records she produces and informs her that the public trustee probably will agree to her becoming Mr L.H.'s guardian. However, there are term deposit certificates that will soon come due, and several bonds are nearing maturity. D. cannot legally instruct the bank to renew the term deposit, nor can she cash the matured savings bonds. The officer therefore takes charge of all Mr L.H.'s finances because he does have the power to deal with the term deposits and bonds.

A review board hearing

Many jurisdictions require that people who have been civilly committed receive a visit from a lawyer or a 'rights' adviser' or, at least, written notification of their legal rights. Mr L.H. is in fact visited by a lawyer. She informs Mr L.H., among other things, of his right to challenge his commitment to hospital before a mental health review board. (In Canada, civil commitments are often challenged before administrative tribunals that do not include a judge but commonly include a lawyer, physician, or other health-care provider and someone who is neither a lawyer nor a provider.) Mr L.H. says that he wants a review board hearing, and he repeatedly tells the lawyer that his son and daughter are stealing from him. The lawyer helps Mr L.H. file an application for a review board hearing and arranges for him to be represented by a lawyer.

Different lawyers take different views of their obligations to manifestly incapable people who wish to contest their civil commitment or to resist a guardianship application. When acting for people who, like Mr L.H., seem manifestly incapable of instructing them, some lawyers do what they believe to be in their client's best interests and will not necessarily follow their instructions. Other lawyers, like Mr L.H.'s, think that by disregarding clients' instructions in civil commitment or guardianship cases they unfairly prejudge their clients' competency – the very issue that the proceedings are to decide authoritatively. Moreover, in some places the law or rules of professional conduct explicitly require lawyers not to prejudge the issue of their clients' competency. Mr L.H.'s lawyer considers herself bound by her client's instructions to challenge vigorously the civil commitment. Among other things, she will make certain that the psychiatrist followed the rules when he committed Mr L.H. as an involuntary patient. She is also concerned by Mr L.H.'s allegations of theft. Although she knows that these may be delusions, she has no proof that they are – his wandering (a summary of the events leading to his committal is contained in the committal form) might have been a pathetic attempt to seek help. Mr L.H. is entitled to make his allegations at a review board hearing, and she will help him do so. D. learns of the impending hearing from Dr B., who will represent himself at the hearing. He will bear the onus of proving that, on a balance of probabilities, Mr L.H.'s civil commitment is justified. In the United States a higher standard of proof – clear and convincing evidence – must often be met to justify a civil commitment, and even in Canada it is sometimes said that the standard for justifying a civil commitment is an 'enhanced' one, that is, somewhat higher than that applied to ordinary civil proceedings. Dr B. tells D. that she will have to testify about Mr L.H.'s wandering to prove that his illness exposes him to a risk of serious bodily harm.

The hearing is held in a boardroom at the hospital. Present are the three members of the review board. One of them is a lawyer, who acts as the board's chairman; one is a psychiatrist; the third is a business woman who views her participation on such panels as a form of public service. Mr L.H., Mr L.H.'s lawyer, Mr L.H.'s psychiatrist, and D. are also present. So is a reporter who will keep a verbatim record of everything that is said at the hearing, and who will prepare a typewritten transcript if anyone brings an appeal from the board's decision.

Dr B. opens his case by giving the board a short outline of the case and presenting a report he has prepared on Mr L.H. All Mr L.H.'s hospital records have previously been made available to Mr L.H.'s lawyer for her to review, as has a copy of Dr B.'s report. The psychiatrist tells the board that, in his opinion, Mr L.H. is suffering from a progressive dementia (possibly Alzheimer's disease) that is quite advanced and that has rendered him almost wholly incapable of making decisions for himself. He also tells the board that in the hospital, as at home, Mr L.H. has demonstrated a propensity to wander, and he must be kept under constant supervision. As well, Mr L.H. is subject to delusions. Mr L.H.'s lawyer cross-examines the psychiatrist. She suggests that D. is stealing from Mr L.H., who wandered from home in a vain attempt to seek help. The psychiatrist answers that Mr L.H.'s memory is so impaired that he would not know if anyone was stealing from him and that false accusations of this kind are very common in demented people.

D. then gives her evidence. She describes her father's deterioration, his persistent accusations of theft, and his wandering, including the incident that led to his hospitalization. Mr L.H.'s lawyer is now quite certain that Mr L.H.'s accusations are false, but still feels a duty to question D. directly about Mr L.H.'s finances. She asks D. whether she has ever stolen from him. D. explains how her father's finances are organized and denies any wrongdoing.

Finally, Mr L.H. testifies. Mr L.H. accuses his daughter of theft, but he cannot say what she has stolen from him. He denies having wandered from home. After a few minutes on the witness stand his speech becomes increasingly disjointed. Ultimately, he appears to have lost all consciousness of where he is or why he is there. The chairman gently thanks Mr L.H. for his help. After Mr L.H.'s performance neither the doctor nor the lawyer feel the need to make any argument to the board; the outcome of the hearing is evident. The board members leave the room for five minutes to confer on their decision and return to announce that they have upheld Mr L.H.'s civil commitment.

Guardianship

Their lawyer has, on D. and S.'s instructions, prepared a guardianship application. The public trustee is acting as Mr L.H.'s lawyer on the application. D. and S.'s lawyer has prepared an affidavit for Dr B. to sign. This affidavit will ultimately be presented to the judge, who will decide whether or not to appoint a guardian for Mr L.H. An affidavit is a document by which a person makes statements of fact or opinion and swears to their truth, either on oath or affirmation, before a person who has the lawful authority to administer an oath or affirmation (usually a lawyer). Affidavits are, among other things, a means of presenting sworn evidence to a judge. The lawyer also prepares an affidavit for the family's physician to sign, and one each for D. and S. The reason for preparing multiple affidavits is that, in general, evidence from more than one person – commonly, two medical professionals and a family member – is required to obtain guardianship. As a further safeguard, the evidence that each person gives must supplement, rather than merely repeat, the evidence that others have provided. Thus, each person involved in seeking a guardianship application will often have to swear out an affidavit that states facts of which he or she is personally aware, and his or her own opinion that guardianship is necessary.

D. and S. will together become the committee of Mr L.H.'s person and estate. In this way, one will always be available to act for Mr L.H. if the other is not. They agree that Mr L.H.'s money should be left in Canada Savings Bonds and term deposit certificates, and that enough money will be kept in a joint bank account to pay for his care in a nursing home. They will be required to keep financial records for Mr L.H.'s money. The necessary forms will be prepared for them by the lawyer's office; they will be similar to records that the executor of an estate must keep, and many law offices have established procedures for the expeditious administration of estates.

The lawyer prepares a plan of financial management for the judge's approval. The public trustee has seen a copy of the proposed plan and will file a document with the court saying that she consents to the appointment of D. and S. as Mr L.H.'s guardians, on the terms that they have proposed. The lawyer appears in court before a judge who has read the affidavits and other materials and who does not require Mr L.H. to appear before him. The judge is convinced that Mr L.H. meets the legal test of mental incompetency and requires a guardian; he signs an order appointing D. and S. the committee of Mr L.H.'s person and estate. They now have the power to choose Mr L.H.'s place of residence, and they will transfer him from the psychiatric hospital to a nursing home as soon as a bed is available for him. They will also have the power to manage Mr L.H.'s estate as soon as they file with the court a bond to guarantee the proper handling of his assets.

Summary

1 Guardianship If an assessment may lead to a guardianship application, has the assessor weighed the risks of guardianship against the risks of going without it?

2 New laws The fact that the guardianship laws to be applied are modern, and provide significant protection for individual liberty, in no way lessens the onus on an assessor to provide a thorough, fair, and comprehensive assessment.

3 Justifying guardianship In general, guardianship should be viewed as a measure of last resort and should be imposed only when it conforms to an incompetent person's previously expressed competent wish, or when the risks associated with not appointing a guardian are grave.

4 Principles of assessment As a general rule, the principles of informal assessment, outlined in chapter 4, and those governing formal assessment (chapter 5) should be followed in making any decision to seek an assessment that may lead to a guardianship order and in performing the assessment itself.

CHAPTER SEVEN

Planning for incompetency

Too often competency assessment is considered solely in relation to the imposition of guardianship. This lends it an unfortunately negative cast; it may seem useful only to distinguish people for whom guardianship is an unavoidable necessity from those for whom it is not. Yet competency assessment can also play a very positive role – especially if the assessors (both formal and informal) have some awareness of the various informal practices and legal mechanisms by which one person may voluntarily give another the power to make decisions on his or her behalf. Assessors who have this knowledge can often help partially incompetent people design a scheme for substitute decision making that is proportional to the extent of their incompetency. Competency assessment can be used to locate the least-restrictive form of care that offers an adequate degree of protection to an incompetent person.

This chapter identifies alternatives to guardianship. Assessors who are aware of these alternatives may sometimes convert the competency assessment of a person who is obviously in some measure impaired, but who is willing to accept another's help, into an assessment of the person's competency to enter into some voluntary arrangement for a substitute decision maker. Such voluntary arrangements (for example, a durable power of attorney) often will delay or entirely forestall the need to resort to guardianship.

This chapter is also intended to serve a different group of people. More and more North Americans now bear the responsibility of caring for aged and ill relatives or have witnessed the decline of a friend or relative. For them the indignities and difficulties that attend the care of people who have not planned for the possibility of mental incompetency have a concrete immediacy. So too has the desirability of planning for the possibility of their own eventual incompetence. Others who have read this book may wish to plan so that they will receive the kind of care that this book advocates, should they become incompetent. Still others may simply wish to avoid ever being subjected to guardianship. Mature people seek to come to terms with the reality of their eventual decline and death. In the past, sober people, aware of their human frailty, have provided for it by making a will that disposes of their property and provides for the protection of their dependents (a testamentary will). In the present, such people may also wish to plan for the possibility that they will become mentally incompetent, and this chapter is addressed to them.

The first part of this chapter describes the informal practices, and the common legal devices, by which people may address the problems of the mentally incompetent. But this is not a self-help book. The discussion does not cover every relevant practice or legal mechanism, and those devices that are considered are discussed only in outline, omitting many details. This chapter is no substitute for the advice of a knowledgable local lawyer.

The second part of this chapter considers some of the advantages and disadvantages of commonly used legal mechanisms for substitute decision making, and some techniques that can be used to overcome or minimize those disadvantages. Again, this information is very general and far from comprehensive. This part of the chapter serves two goals. First, to supply people with the information they need to begin thinking about the kind of plan that they might wish to make for themselves, or that they might wish to encourage another, partially incompetent person to make. Second, to supply assessors with background information about the nature of some commonly used legal devices, so that they can grasp the issues that arise in assessing competency to perform legal acts such as making a power of attorney or a will.

The third part of this chapter consists of three assessments of competency to perform legal acts. The law sets its own standards for competency to perform legal acts, and those standards, although broadly similar in form, vary quite considerably from jurisdiction to jurisdiction. These sample assessments illustrate some common problems and a generally applicable approach to their resolution – one that can easily be adapted to incorporate the standards for competency in different jurisdictions. In fine, this chapter is not about the law as such, but rather about the relationship between law and competency assessment; it is intended to illustrate a sound, general approach that can be adapted to the laws of different places.

Why plan?

With proper planning, people can assure themselves that a substitute decision maker of their own choosing will be available to them if they become incompetent, and at the same time they can minimize the costs of obtaining such assistance. Most important, by making their own plans for care in the event of incompetency, they can ensure that if they become incompetent their special needs, concerns, or wishes will be known to, and honored by, their substitute decision makers. Moreover, by making such plans people may ease the burden that their infirmities impose on others and forestall or prevent the need to resort to more intrusive legal mechanisms for substitute decision making, principally guardianship.

Self-planned care often has advantages of economy, flexibility, and speed over guardianship. But for many people who plan for their own care or protection these are secondary considerations. More often people derive considerable satisfaction from the knowledge that they have provided for their own needs in the event of incompetency. This satisfaction seems to have two powerful, and in some measure contradictory, sources. First, people think of planning as a means of extending their independence and self-control. For example, a plan may provide for partial incompetency in a way that the applicable guardianship law does not. Or it may determine the circumstances in which an incompetent person will live (providing for care outside an institution like a nursing home). However, there does seem to be a measure of self-deception in the idea that by planning people can somehow extend their autonomy beyond a point where nature will have otherwise deprived them of it. The reality is that some measure of incompetency, like death, is likely to afflict everyone sooner or later. Planning for the possibility of incompetency is a way of coming to grips with this reality. It is a kind of self-overcoming that brings with it the satisfaction that every kind of self-mastery does. In both practical and emotional terms, therefore, considerable advantages are to be derived from planning for incompetency.

Why encourage others to plan?

In the chapter on guardianship, and elsewhere in the book, those who

provide care to partially incompetent people, and competency assessors, have been urged to favor voluntary measures like the power of
attorney over involuntary measures like guardianship. This chapter is
intended to reinforce the point. The principle of the least-restrictive
alternative requires that involuntary measures be considered as
measures of last resort, to be used only for people who are unable or
unwilling to plan for their own protection. As well, plans for substitute
decision making that people have made for themselves often have
other advantages over plans that are imposed on them. The process of
obtaining guardianship is often slow and expensive and can be humiliating to both the incompetent person and his or her family. Moreover,
the process of imposing care on a person who resists it may establish
an adversarial relationship between an incompetent person and his or
her guardian that makes the process of providing care miserable for all
involved. Voluntary or consensual care is preferable to involuntary care
whenever either is sufficient to meet an incompetent person's needs.

Working things out

It should not be assumed that a formal legal response is the only, or
the best, imaginable way to meet the needs of a partially incompetent
person. Although it is often necessary to appoint a substitute decision
maker who can immediately begin to act, one goal of planning is to
avoid or delay this eventuality. Often people who are only partially and
mildly incompetent, and who can make most of their own day-to-day
decisions, are able to work their problems out one at a time without
the assistance of a substitute decision maker. An informal competency
assessment will often identify such people. For example, an assessment
may reveal that a person cannot write checks but can review a bank
statement; rather than take control of his or her financial affairs a
friend or relative might arrange to have the person's bills automatically
paid from his or her bank account. Or, another example, a person
may have difficulty purchasing groceries during the winter months and
so be at risk of harm from improper diet. Rather than jumping to the
conclusion that the person needs to live in a protected environment
where meals are supplied, a concerned friend or relative might
arrange to have the person's groceries delivered by a local store. Working things out in practice means that people should seek and take
advantage of all available assistance for themselves or others as a substitute for, or an adjunct to, more formal legal responses.

Although one purpose of working things out is to avoid reliance on a substitute decision maker, it is important to recognize that a substitute decision maker may (and often should) be appointed in advance of need. Simply put, good planning gives people – especially those who are already partially incompetent – an opportunity to choose a substitute decision maker who may never have to exercise his or her powers. Even when it is possible to work things out, people should consider the possibility that at some point it may no longer be possible to do so. The appointment of a substitute decision maker is like purchasing insurance – people do it hoping to never call on it. As a general rule, it is particularly important for people who are partially incompetent (or who, like those suffering from the active symptoms of Alzheimer's disease, are highly likely to become incompetent) to select and instruct a substitute decision maker.

Planning for financial incompetency

It is common for people to become unable to manage their own financial affairs although they are capable of managing other aspects of their lives. As well, many incapable people have very few assets and only a single source of income. In such circumstances an adequate plan of care for an incompetent person may involve little more than obtaining the power to gain access to that person's bank account or pension benefits. There are a number of relatively informal, and widely available legal devices by which such arrangements can be made. These may be used either as an alternative or an adjunct to a more comprehensive plan for substitute decision making. They include joint bank accounts, bank powers of attorney, and representative payees who receive and manage benefits on behalf of an incompetent person. A more complex approach is to establish a trust.

Joint bank accounts

The contents of a joint bank account are owned by more than one person, each of whom may withdraw or deposit funds into it. A joint bank account may or may not have a right of survivorship attached to it. If the account incorporates this right then, if one joint owner dies, ownership of the entire account is automatically transferred to the surviving owner or owners. Whether an account involves this right will depend on the banking forms used to establish it and also on local laws. A joint account may be used to provide for incompetency, since one owner may use the money in the account on behalf of another owner who has become incompetent. Joint accounts thus can be an especially useful planning device for spouses, particularly those who already pool their assets in a common account. When incompetency arises suddenly and without warning (as, for example, with a person who has suffered a head injury in an automobile accident) an incompetent person's dependents may be left without enough money for their immediate needs. A joint bank account to which one or more of a person's dependents has access is one way to avoid such predicaments. The major drawback of joint accounts is the absence of any formal mechanisms to check the other owner, acting as a substitute decision maker (such as checks that may apply to guardians) or of well-known and recognized rules of conduct that the other owner must obey (as with trustees). Moreover, in the absence of a trusted friend or relative to be joint owner, the joint bank account is simply not a useful planning device.

Bank power of attorney

Like a joint account, a bank power of attorney is a means of giving one person lawful access to another's bank account. It is a limited form of power of attorney by which a principal gives his or her agent the right to deal with the principal's bank account. Unlike a joint account, a bank power of attorney does not involve a transfer of ownership or a right of survivorship – the bank account remains the sole property of the principal. Many financial institutions recognize that their customers have many reasons for allowing others access to their accounts. At the same time these institutions are often reluctant to accept individualized durable powers of attorneys, for they fear possible liability if they wrongly interpret the power and so wrongly grant access to an account. To solve the problem many institutions offer their customers a standard form of power of attorney that they may execute for the purpose of granting another access to their accounts. The advantages of a bank power of attorney are that it offers more certain access to the account than an individualized power of attorney does, without requiring a transfer of ownership in the account as joint ownership does. As well, the bank power of attorney offers an incompetent person the protection of a principal-agent relationship. People who execute multiple powers of attorney (for example, a durable power of attorney for finances and a bank power of attorney) *must* seek the advice of a lawyer so that the separate documents do not inadvertently cancel one another out or result in confusion about the extent of an attorney's authority.

Representative payees

Poverty is unfortunately common among the elderly or disabled, many of whom subsist on pensions or disability benefits. Some benefit or pension plans permit a person (a *representative* or a *representative payee*) to apply to receive and administer an incompetent person's benefits. If an incompetent person receives public benefits of some kind, the substitute decider (even one who holds legal authority to manage the person's finances) may have to take special steps to receive and administer them. If a pension or disability benefit is a person's sole or major source of income, and if the person's incompetency is limited to financial decision making, a representative payee may be the least-restrictive form of substitute decision making.

The trust

A trust is a legal arrangement by which one person (called, depending on local laws and practices, the grantor or settlor) gives money or property to a person or persons (the trustee or trustees) who hold and use it on behalf of themselves or others (the beneficiaries), subject to the relevant local laws and to any directions or restrictions that the settlor has imposed upon them. Some trusts are established by wills, and these are called testamentary trusts. Other trusts are established by people during their lifetimes and these are called *inter vivos* or living trusts. A settlor may be his or her own beneficiary, and a trust does not cease to operate only because a beneficiary (or, if properly planned, an executor) becomes incompetent to manage financial matters. Thus, people may use the trust to plan for the possibility of their incompetency. Such people may establish a living trust and select a trustee who, if the settlor becomes incompetent, will oversee it and make financial decisions on the settlor's behalf. A settlor has great flexibility in determining when the trust will become active and (subject to applicable legislation) in determining what powers the trustees will have. Some people, for example, establish as a 'dry' or 'standby' trust (that is, a trust that initially holds no, or very little, money or property) but arrange to have funds transferred into the trust if they become financially incompetent.

Many precedents exist for the creation of trusts, and long-standing rules guide the conduct of trustees and protect beneficiaries. Trusts are extremely flexible devices, and the terms of their establishment may be varied to meet many individual needs and to provide for many contingencies. However, it is sometimes expensive to comply with the formalities of establishing and maintaining a trust, and they are often unsuitable devices for people who have little property and few assets. The principal disadvantage of a trust is that it is only a vehicle for financial planning and does not answer the need for substitute personal decision making. Nonetheless it can be a valuable element of a more comprehensive plan which involves as well the use of a power of attorney, a subject that is considered below.

Wills

The relatively informal devices discussed above may suffice to provide for people whose incompetency is relatively minor, or who have few assets. But for many people they will be useful only as one element of a more comprehensive and sophisticated plan for their own protection. As a general rule, the first step in executing such a plan, for a person who has not already done so, is to execute a will.

A will is a formal legal document, usually (but not always) drafted by a lawyer who holds it in his or her confidential possession pending the will-maker's death. By their wills people determine the disposition of their property after their deaths. A male person who makes a will is called a testator and a female person who does so is called a testatrix. A gift made in a will is called a bequest or legacy, and the person who receives the gift is called a beneficiary or legatee. A will also designates a person (or people) to manage the deceased person's estate; if male this person is called an executor and if female an executrix. In this book, however, both male and female will-makers are called testators, and both male and female estate-managers are called executors. An executor is a trustee, which means that he or she has legal possession of the deceased's property on behalf of the beneficiaries to whom it ultimately belongs. The executor must generally have the will formally recognized as a legally binding instrument (the process of doing so is usually called probate), pay the deceased's taxes and debts, and then distribute the estate's assets to the beneficiaries.

The will as part of a competency plan

It may seem strange to think of a will as part of a plan for incompetency: wills speak only after someone's death, and incompetency planning addresses the needs of the living. But this impression, although understandable, is erroneous.

1   When people prepare a will they must decide whom they trust to act as their executors. Thus, the preparation of a will is also often an ideal moment to select the person (or persons) whom an individual wishes to act as substitute decision maker in the event of need.

2   A very common goal of will making is to protect the testator's dependents. But incompetency can deprive dependents of protection as effectively as death can, so the preparation of a will without an accompanying plan for incompetency is an incomplete exercise.

3   People must often consult a lawyer to prepare their wills, just as they must often consult them to prepare a plan for incompetency. It is often more convenient and less expensive to prepare a plan for incompetency when a will is being prepared than it is to prepare both plans separately.

4   People often have strong feeling about the disposition of their property on their deaths. But when people wait too long to make their wills they run the risk of becoming incompetent to do so. Moreover, when people who are partially competent make wills (especially unconventional wills that disappoint the expectations of some of their friends or relatives) their capacity to make a will, or the authenticity of the will they make, may be challenged after their deaths. To be sure that their own wishes will be followed, and to avoid needless litigation that may deplete their estates, people should think of a will as a precautionary step in a plan for incompetency.

Testamentary capacity

The law has its own test of the mental capacity to make a will (the technical term is 'testamentary capacity'). Although the definition of testamentary capacity differs from place to place, its general outline is broadly similar in most North American jurisdictions. To have the capacity to make a will a person must have the abilities to:

1 Understand the nature of the legal act that he or she is performing.

2 Identify all of his or her property.

3 Identify all those whom he or she would ordinarily, because of family connection, dependence, affection or moral obligation, consider as potential beneficiaries.

4 Use all the above information in independently deciding who will receive what part of his or her property.

In the United States the law often refers to a person who has testamentary capacity as being of 'sound mind' or of 'sound and disposing mind.'

Partial incompetency and undue influence

A will normally is invalid if made by a person who did not have testamentary capacity. But even a will made by a person who has testamentary capacity may be invalid if it was made by a person who was under another's 'undue influence,' that is, if the will does not reflect its maker's authentic and independent wishes, but rather those of someone who unduly imposed themselves on the will-maker. Often people who are partially incompetent are, for a variety of reasons, unusually open to others' manipulation. When people urge someone else who is incompetent, or becoming so, to make a will, they must consider whether the person has testamentary capacity and also be careful to avoid exercising an undue influence over the will-making. More pointedly stated, people who urge others to make a will, even if they have perfectly legitimate reasons for doing so, must be careful not to become so involved in the process that they render the resulting will open to challenge, if not invalid.

The precise definition of undue influence varies from place to place, and undue influence may arise in a myriad of situations. A useful general rule is that a person who wishes to discuss will-making with another person should (*especially* if the other person is frail, incapacitated, or dependent upon them) seek legal advice *before* initiating these discussions. Although it may be entirely proper to suggest to an incompetent person that he or she make a will, it is generally best to encourage him or her to seek information about wills from a lawyer, or from some other neutral third party.

Powers of attorney

A power of attorney is a legal document by which one person (who, depending on local laws and practices, may be called the creator, donor, grantor, or principal) appoints another person (who, again depending on local laws and practices, may be called the donee, grantee, agent, or attorney-in-fact) to make decisions regarding personal care, or finances, or both, on his or her behalf. In this book the person who makes a power of attorney is called the principal, and the person who is given the power to make substitute decisions is called the agent. Generally put, an agent is a person who has the legal power to exercise the legal rights or powers of another person who has appointed him or her to do so. A real estate agent, for example, has the legal authority to offer property for sale that does not belong to him or her.

The powers that the agent receives may be adjusted to match the principal's present or anticipated needs, and they can range from broad and complete control of a person's affairs to much more limited and specific authority. For example, a person with Alzheimer's disease might empower someone to make all of his or her financial and medical decisions. A person who is mentally competent, but blind, might execute a power of attorney that merely gives his or her agent access to a safety deposit box. A power of attorney that is used to plan for incompetency will often give the agent complete, or near complete, control of the donor's property in the event of the donor's incompetence. In this way, the agent is able to cope with unforeseen or unforeseeable contingencies as they arise.

Enduring powers of attorney

Powers of attorney originated as useful commercial devices. For example, an importer might use a power of attorney to give an agent at the ship docks the authority to execute the documents necessary to clear the goods through customs. In many places powers of attorney automatically became invalid if the principal became mentally incompetent. This rule made sense in a commercial setting, where a principal would likely expect to supervise his or her agent. But the rule of automatic termination meant that people could not use powers of attorney as a flexible, inexpensive, and expeditious means of appointing substitute decision makers to act for them if they became incompetent. As a result, many North American and other jurisdictions passed new legislation, establishing a power of attorney that remains valid even if the principal becomes mentally incompetent. Such powers of attorney are often called enduring or durable powers of attorney, to distinguish them from powers of attorney that become invalid if their maker ceases to be mentally competent.

The enduring or durable power of attorney is a widely available and extremely useful device for appointing a substitute decision maker. Many lawyers advise their clients to use it.

Springing powers of attorney

Appointing a substitute decision maker in advance of need is a kind of insurance against incompetency. But people who make enduring powers of attorney often want some assurance that their agent will not act prematurely, that is, while they are still competent. One way to do this is to have a trusted person (often a lawyer) hold the power of attorney under instructions to release it only when necessary. Another way, offering still greater protection, is to specify in the power of attorney the circumstances in which the agent may begin to act. This kind of power, which becomes valid only when certain events have happened or specified conditions are satisfied, is called a springing power of attorney.

A springing power of attorney 'springs' to life when it is needed but not before. For example, a person might specify that his or her power of attorney becomes effective only when two physicians have certified in writing that he or she is financially incapable. This person might also designate the assessors, or classes of assessors (for example, geriatricians or psychiatrists) from whom the assessment must be obtained. In some places the law explicitly recognizes the validity of springing powers of attorney, but even in the absence of such explicit approval it is often possible to make them.

Health-care powers of attorney

Durable powers of attorney were first used to provide for financial matters. But people increasingly demanded an inexpensive and flexible means of appointing and instructing someone to make or execute decisions about their personal care in the event of incompetency. As a result many American states have passed, and many Canadian provinces have either passed or are actively considering the passage of, laws that explicitly recognize what are in effect durable powers of attorney for medical decisions. These are sometimes called medical-care or health-care powers of attorney, or health-care proxies. In other states and provinces the laws do not explicitly approve of such devices but they have been recognized by the courts or are accepted in practice. In still other states it is generally accepted that the legislation that recognizes general durable powers of attorney is sufficiently broad to include health-care (or personal decision) powers of attorney. In Canada the validity of such devices is often unclear, but the situation is rapidly changing for the better. At present, though, many Canadian lawyers appear to think that a durable or enduring power of attorney may be applied only to financial decision making, and some provincial statutes explicitly restrict the application of durable powers of attorney to the management of finances or property.

Health-care powers of attorney distinguished from living wills

Many American states have passed laws that allow people to express wishes about the treatment they want to receive or forego in the final stages of their lives. These are often called Natural Death Acts, after the California law that was the first of its kind. Among other things, these laws allow people whose deaths are imminent to reject some kinds of life-sustaining treatment. Some, but not all, of these laws also allow people to appoint a proxy or agent to express, interpret, or make health-care decisions for them. Living wills govern only end-of-life care, and the statutes governing them often limit the kind of treatment that a person may lawfully refuse: for example, some laws prevent people from refusing food or water. By contrast, powers of attorney for health care may provide for medical substitute decision making in general and not only for decisions in connection with end-of-life care.

Advance directives: living wills

The term 'advance directive' encompasses the entire range of devices by which people who are competent at the time may issue instructions regarding the personal care, including medical treatment, they wish to receive if they become incompetent. Special considerations arise in relation to the making of decisions regarding medical care in advance of need, especially when those decisions govern the treatment people wish to receive or forego if they are dying and incompetent to make their own treatment decisions.

Advance directives may be usefully subdivided into two general types – proxy and instruction directives. A proxy directive names the person whom a currently competent person wants to have act as a substitute decision maker in the event of incompetency. It may or may not incorporate specific instructions that the substitute decision maker should follow. In contrast, an instruction directive incorporates specific instructions that are to be followed in the event of the maker's incompetency. Many directives both express specific instructions or wishes and name a proxy to make decisions regarding matters that are not explicitly dealt with in the directive.

The best-known and most often discussed form of advance directive is commonly called a living will. A living will is a legal device by which people may indicate their desire to receive, or to forego, various kinds of life-sustaining care in the event that they require such care and are incompetent to make their own decisions regarding it. Typically, living wills express instructions regarding such treatments as tube-feeding, the use of artificial breathing machines (ventilators) or kidney dialysis machines, and electrical or chemical resuscitation following a heart attack or stroke. Generally, advance directives distinguish the circumstances in which the instruction is binding. For example, people often want to receive a particular treatment (say, resuscitation following a heart attack) if there is a reasonable chance that it will restore them to active, independent life, but do not want to receive it if it will merely prolong the process of their dying. The legal effect of a living will varies from place to place, as do the requirements governing who may make one and the range of treatments that it can relate to.

The general trend in North America is to expand both the right to make advance directives and the kinds of decisions that can lawfully be incorporated in them. But the laws that apply to advance directives vary, sometimes significantly, from place to place. Even more than in other areas of concern, in planning for medical decision making it is imperative to seek advice from a lawyer and a health-care professional who are aware of commonly used and recognized forms of advance directives, the procedures that govern the making of a legally valid one, and any restrictions that the local law imposes on their contents. There is a plethora of excellent materials on the subject of living wills, and people who are thinking of making one should also ask a knowledgeable professional to recommend a publication that deals with the laws of their own jurisdiction.

Although advance directives are an essential part of planning for incompetency they are no panacea. This caveat applies with special force to living wills, the advantages of which seem to have attracted more notice than the potential disadvantages have. The following discussion is intended, in part, to redress this imbalance, but it is not designed to tell people whether they should, or should not, make a living will. That is a decision that turns both on individual circumstances and local laws, and so it should be made in consultation with a local lawyer or health-care professional. Rather, this discussion is aimed primarily at people who are already thinking of making a living will, and it is designed to help them clarify their thoughts about why they propose to make one and to begin thinking about the form that it might take.

By their living wills people may gain some measure of assurance that they will receive the kind of treatment that they want, and be spared treatments that they do not want, in the final stages of their lives. It is, in other words, a means by which people may seek to receive while dying and incompetent the care that they would choose to receive if they were dying and competent to make treatment decisions. A living will may also sometimes spare the family, friends, or medical caregivers of a dying and incompetent person some of the agony that goes with making life-or-death decisions on behalf of a person whose own wishes are unknown. One other reason for making a living will may be mentioned. Living wills are seen by some as a legitimate way to avoid the unwarranted expenditure of scarce health-care dollars on end-of-life care, and some altruistic individuals may execute one to this end.

Properly handled, the making of a living will (and other forms of advance directive) will often involve discussion between its maker and his or her family, friends, spiritual advisor, or physician (or other health-care providers). Indeed, the process of discussion, clarification of thought and feeling, and communication of wishes that goes with the making of a living will may be as valuable as the resulting document is.

It is not always as easy as people think it is to make a living will or other advance directive that accurately forecasts the care or treatment that the maker would accept or reject in particular circumstances if competent to do so. The making of a directive involves casting the mind into the future, assessing one's likely wishes or desires in the face of some imagined calamity. It is one thing for people to engage in this imaginative process when the nature, and even the likelihood, of the imagined calamity can be forecast with some accuracy, and quite another when such accurate prediction is impossible. Thus, it is one thing for a person who is actively suffering from some fatal illness or disease, such as AIDS or lung cancer, to make a living will, and another thing altogether for a healthy person who is making judgments entirely in the abstract to do so. The problem is particularly acute when people make judgments based on a present assessment of their likely 'quality of life' in the face of some future contingency; often, what a healthy person views as a terrible or insupportable life does not seem so to a person who is actually enduring it. As well, thoughts and feelings about end-of-life care often change as people age. Of course it is possible to accommodate these changes by revising a living will at regular intervals; indeed, people who make living wills should reconsider and revise them at regular intervals. But such revision cannot entirely overcome the possibility that a person will become incompetent and have his or her treatment determined by an out-of-date living will.

Other difficulties arise from the use of preprinted forms to make living wills or from professionals who draft living wills by precedent and without adequate attention to the maker's individual needs. Even when forms or precedents provide a reasonable array of choices, and an opportunity for the makers to express their own unusual choices or wishes (and not all forms and precedents are adequate in this regard), they often cannot capture the entire range of considerations that people take into account when actually making decisions about their health care. More simply, it is often difficult to draft a living will that accurately reflects the decisions that an incompetent person would make were he or she competent to do so.

There are two general points to bear in mind for anyone making a living will. First, living wills are no substitute for discussion between their makers and the people who must express and implement the decisions recorded in them. As a practical matter, a living will can be effective only if its existence is known to those who are expected to act on it. The making of a living will thus should be treated as an opportunity for the maker to reflect on his or her own thoughts, feelings, and wishes regarding death and dying, and also for discussion with others who may be affected by the living will. Second, the process of assessing competency to make an advance directive has received surprisingly little attention. A full treatment of such assessment is, for various reasons, beyond the scope of this book. The principal reason is that only recently have people begun to consider the peculiar difficulties that beset the assessment of a person's present ability to make a medical decision that will take effect in the future and that (in contrast to a will governing the disposition of property) may have very significant implications for its maker during his or her lifetime. A related and weighty reason is the difficulty of sorting through the implications for competency assessment of the different kinds of living wills. Thus, the criteria and procedure of assessment will differ according to local laws, the condition of the living will's maker, whether the living will incorporates or does not incorporate a proxy appointment, and the foreseeability and imminence of the circumstances addressed in the living will.

The likelihood of a living will actually being followed will depend not only on making it known to others, but also on the degree of faith that those others have in it as an accurate expression of the maker's competent wishes. This is another reason why people should discuss their reasons for making a living will with those whom they expect to follow it. It is also a reason why professionals who assist people in making a living will should, at a minimum, while making the living will document the process that led up to its creation and especially any observations relevant to an assessment of the maker's competence. Like lawyers who help people make testamentary wills, all those who help people make living wills have a responsibility – if not legal then certainly moral – to document adequately the competency of those who make them as a safeguard against future challenges.

Summary

When people plan for the care of an incompetent person, or when a partially incompetent person plans for his or her own care, they must first decide what kind of care is called for in the circumstances. Fully competent people may be able to do this themselves – that is, they may look ahead, forecast their likely future needs, and plan to have them met according to the general principles outlined in this book. Even so, they may want to seek help from family, friends, financial and medical advisers, and others. For people who are already partially incompetent, such help in planning is almost certain to be needed. Perhaps even a formal assessment will be required. The principles outlined in previous chapters, relating to present disabilities, apply equally to planning for any future incompetence. The first rule is still to base care on a proper assessment; needs must be identified before they can be supplied. A primary goal of such assessment is to locate the least-intrusive form of care that will adequately protect an incompetent person.

An adequate plan for incompetency, even one made by someone who is able to make many or all of his or her own decisions, will almost always involve the appointment and instruction of a substitute decision maker or makers. These agents will have broad powers to make decisions on the maker's behalf should he or she become substantially or wholly incompetent. Often the process of assessment will involve educating a person about the range of voluntary devices open to him or her and about their respective advantages and disadvantages. The following section of this chapter is a guide to some of the relevant considerations in selecting and using legal devices to plan for incompetency.

General concerns in planning for substitute decision making

Risk

Like all relationships in which one person is dependent on another, substitute decision making carries an inherent risk of abuse. The term 'abuse' in this context covers a range of actions, from negligence or incompetence in the management of the maker's finances to outright theft, and from overprotectiveness to physical neglect or actual violence. The risk arises not solely from the relationship of dependency, but also because many self-designed arrangements for substitute decision making are devised and executed privately without notice to any disinterested third party who can monitor the behavior of a substitute decider. There are, however, steps that people can take to lessen substantially the risk of abuse associated with self-designed arrangements for substitute decision making.

This part of the chapter is obviously relevant to competent people who are thinking of devising a plan for their own care in the event of incompetency. It may also be useful, in two ways, to competency assessors. First, assessors who discuss with partially incompetent people the possibility of selecting and appointing a substitute decision maker must have some knowledge of the issues that those agents are likely to have to consider. Second, assessments of the ability to perform legal acts (including the making of an enduring power of attorney) often focus on the maker's ability to understand the risks associated with the decisions that they make. Thus, an assessor must have some appreciation of what those risks are before he or she can plan and perform an adequate assessment.

Choosing an appropriate caregiver

The best way to avoid abuse is to choose an appropriate and trustworthy caregiver. Indeed, when financial affairs are uncomplicated, the primary criteria for choosing an appropriate substitute are his or her trustworthiness and compatibility with the person whom he or she is to protect. But in many instances the substitute decider must have financial acumen in addition to being trustworthy and likeable. For example, the owner of a large business should prefer a substitute decider who has solid financial skills and who is trustworthy over one who has little financial skill and who is unreliable but who is very likeable. In selecting an appropriate substitute decider, the first step should be to assess the kinds of decisions the agent will have to make, and only then ask which person is both trustworthy and able to make them.

If a competency assessment is required, it should examine not only the partially incompetent person's specific disabilities or needs, but also the kind of substitute decider that is required.

Providing assistance to the caregiver

An incompetent person's needs are often manifold, and even the most trustworthy and diligent caregiver may not be able to answer all of them. People should also remember in planning for their own care that they should avoid imposing unreasonable burdens on those who care for them. Often the most desirable substitute decider may be unwilling or unable to assume the entire burden of managing all of another person's affairs. In such a case the appropriate action is not simply to reject the substitute as inappropriate, but rather to consider the possibility of arranging appropriate support for the substitute. For example, a person who is planning for incompetency might retain and train a bookkeeper or an accountant who will, in event of need, also be available to assist a substitute decider. Alternatively, a substitute decider can be given the power and means, and even encouraged, to select and pay assistants of his or her own choice. A third solution is to appoint more than one substitute (say, a trusted friend *and* an attorney as joint agents under a power of attorney), although such arrangements may lead to conflict and expense. Finally, people may appoint different substitutes to manage different parts of their lives. For example, a person might choose his or her spouse to make personal decisions, but an institution (such as a bank or a trust company) to manage finances.

In addition to reducing the burden on a substitute, arrangements like these may build some measure of protection against abuse into voluntary and private arrangements for substitute decision making. For example, people who live in jurisdictions where substitutes are not required to account for their actions might wish to build some kind of accountability into a plan for substitute decision making. They might require an agent under a power of attorney to maintain appropriate records that are subject to a third-party yearly audit, even though local laws impose no such obligation on the agent.

When people arrange for substitute decision making they should consider not only their own capacity and needs, but also the limitations of their chosen substitute deciders.

Alternate caregivers

It sometimes happens that a substitute becomes unable or unwilling to act after the person who appointed him or her becomes incompetent. In such cases, there may be no alternative to restrictive forms of decision making such as guardianship, and an incompetent person thus may come under the control of someone whom he or she would, if competent, reject as a substitute decision maker. This eventuality can be prevented by appointing alternate substitutes. Elderly spouses who appoint one another as substitute deciders are particularly well advised to consider appointing as well an alternate substitute; it is not uncommon for spouses to be simultaneously incompetent at some time during their lives and so unable to care for one another. The risk that a voluntary plan for substitute decision making will fail because the substitute becomes unable or unwilling to act may be reduced, if not overcome, by selecting alternate – or multiple – substitutes.

Who says when? Who says what?

A proper plan for incompetency makes help available only when it is needed and not before, and it should require the help offered to be task-specific. For example, modern guardianship legislation requires that judges limit the powers that they grant to a guardian so that they correspond with the individual person's specific disabilities. A judge applying such modern laws would appoint a guardian to make both financial and personal decisions for a person in the late stages of Alzheimer's disease, but a guardian to make only financial decisions for a stroke victim who can no longer manage his or her complicated financial affairs but who can make his or her own personal decisions. Individuals planning for their own incompetency may wish to impose similar requirements on their substitutes. For example, a person might execute a springing power of attorney that comes to life only after a proper competency assessment has determined that the principal is incompetent.

For some people it will, however, be too onerous, unnecessary, or dangerous to require an assessment before a substitute can begin to act on his or her behalf. This will often be the case, for example, with people who periodically require speedy assistance – among them those suffering from episodic attacks of mania or depression, or schizophrenics who periodically undergo episodes of severe psychosis. Even when substitutes do not need an assessment to tell them that some form of intervention is required, however, they will often benefit by performing an informal assessment to clarify exactly what kind of care to supply. The mere possession of a power is not always a reason to exercise it, or to exercise it to its fullest extent.

Even with the simplest devices in planning for incompetency – devices like a bank power of attorney or joint property that do not require prior competency assessment – it is prudent to discuss with the chosen substitute the provision of task-specific care, and so be assured that the substitute has some idea of what it involves. Indeed, such a discussion, although perhaps not a sufficient guarantee of respectful care, is often a necessary one – people cannot be expected to meet others' expectations unless they know what they are. Although some substitute decision makers are neglectful or abusive, more probably fail to provide good care to an incompetent person only because they do not understand how to do so. Open communication between a substitute and the person who has chosen him or her is an essential part of planning for incompetency.

Assessing competency to perform legal acts: three examples

Some of the most challenging assessment cases involve people who are partially incompetent, but who may still be capable of choosing their own substitute decision maker or of performing other legal acts, such as making a will. The following cases illustrate some of the problems that arise in these kinds of assessments. The cases are *not* meant as accurate or full discussions of relevant legal doctrines, but rather to illustrate how assessments may be tailored to meet both individual circumstances and applicable legal principles.

The first assessment concerns an area (competency to instruct counsel) in which the relevant rules are notoriously vague and applies standards that the Competency Clinic itself has developed. This case does not apply the law as it is, but rather the law as the authors think it should be. The second case concerns testamentary capacity, the general definition of which is substantially similar in all North American jurisdictions, but the details of which differ from place to place. This assessment is based on Canadian legal principles. The third case deals with assessing capacity to execute a power of attorney. The case law on this subject varies dramatically from place to place, and it is impossible to formulate a general rule of broad application. This case example is based on judicial decisions from England and the province of Ontario (in Ontario, soon to be superseded by statute) that render the power of attorney a particularly useful planning device. To repeat a crucial point: these assessments are not intended to illustrate the law, but rather to show how competency assessment and legal doctrine can interact.

Mrs N.L.: Competency to instruct a lawyer

Mrs N.L. suffers from schizophrenia and has recently been abandoned and left destitute by her husband. When she was taken by her social worker to see a lawyer she was barely coherent. Lawyers are generally forbidden to act on the instructions of a mentally incompetent person, and the lawyer whom Mrs N.L. consulted feared that she was incompetent to instruct him. When no one could be found to bring a lawsuit on Mrs N.L.'s behalf, the lawyer arranged for her to have a competency assessment.

What is competency to instruct counsel?

In general a client who instructs a lawyer must understand the nature of the proceedings in which he or she wishes to become involved, and the potential legal and personal consequences of involvement in them. The client must recognize the nature of the dispute, the official and binding character of legal proceedings, and the kinds of decisions that he or she will likely be required to make during them. The client must also appreciate the nature of the authority that he or she gives to her lawyer. Most lawyers seek fairly complete control of the work that they do, and competent people must appreciate the degree of trust that they repose in their lawyers.

Mrs N.L. wishes to receive both financial support and property from her husband. She also wants a divorce. She must understand that divorce means that she will no longer be married to her husband and that they will both be free to marry again if they wish to. She must also understand that these legal proceedings will finally (and perhaps permanently) settle all financial obligations between her and her husband. Her ability to support herself will be an issue in the legal proceedings. She will have to reveal details of her illness to her husband's lawyer, and she may even have to be assessed by a psychiatrist or other health-care professional whom her husband's lawyer will select. As well, her own psychiatrist will probably have to make a report about her that will be given to her husband's lawyer. Ultimately, both Mrs N.L. and her psychiatrist may have to testify at a public trial, although her lawyer thinks that this is very unlikely. Most likely, Mrs N.L.'s lawsuit will be settled out of court. If the lawsuit were to go to trial, and were she to lose, Mrs N.L. could be required to pay her husband's legal costs; it is highly unlikely that this will happen, but her lawyer feels an obligation to inform her of the possibility, especially because it would be so disastrous for her were it to occur. In summary, Mrs N.L. must appreciate that legal proceedings will bring to a close her relationship with her husband, will probably result in her obtaining support and property that she could not otherwise obtain, may expose her to a very small risk of personal liability for her husband's costs, and will almost certainly expose her to the embarrassment of publicly discussing her illness.

The assessment

Mrs N.L.'s competency is to be assessed by the psychiatrist (Dr X.) who has treated her regularly for years. Dr X. has spoken with Mrs N.L.'s lawyer and has a general understanding of the proposed legal proceedings. Mrs N.L. has been given a psychological test and the results are consistent with earlier tests; she is quite intelligent, and her memory is generally good. Her major problems are disordered perception (unless she takes medication she hears voices whose urgings she cannot resist); chronic, general emotional flatness; and, occasionally, overwhelming feelings of hopelessness and despair. Based on the test and past experience, Dr X. is sure that Mrs N.L. can absorb information about her lawsuit. He is concerned, however, that her delusions, or her general emotional state, might deprive her of the ability to exercise judgment: she might, for example, make quixotic decisions because she wrongly thinks that her situation is utterly hopeless and is unprepared to accept information to the contrary. He also fears that she may lack directive ability, which means the ability to formulate and express instructions that others will follow: she sometimes has extreme difficulty in bringing herself to make even very simple decisions. In the end, Dr X. thinks that Mrs N.L.'s lawyer is right to be concerned about her competency to instruct him and that a formal assessment of her competency to instruct counsel is indeed necessary.

Dr X. has by no means concluded that Mrs N.L. is incompetent, but he has used his knowledge of her to narrow the scope of his formal competency assessment. Dr X. knows that he cannot infer the existence of incompetency merely from the presence of a major mental illness and that Mrs N.L. is entitled to a fair and task-specific assessment.

Before he begins the assessment he must obtain Mrs N.L.'s consent. Dr X. explains to Mrs N.L. that their next few sessions together will be different from their usual ones. He tells her that her lawyer has asked him to explore Mrs N.L.'s ability to instruct a lawyer. He also tells her that he might decide that she cannot instruct a lawyer, and if he does so she might not be allowed to make decisions about taking legal proceedings against her husband. Finally, he tells her that he knows that she has been very upset by her husband's conduct and that he will continue to help her in any way that he can even if she does not want him to assess her. He then asks her to repeat (in her own words) what he has just said to her. She accurately recounts what he has said, and she says that she wants to take her husband to court if she can and would like to have the assessment.

Having secured Mrs N.L.'s consent, the doctor proceeds with the assessment. He will have to move very slowly and in stages. Any woman would be extremely upset if her husband abandoned her and left her destitute, and Mrs N.L. is unusually sensitive to stress; when she is upset she tends to become disoriented and her speech becomes disjointed and halting. She is at present in such a state, but Dr X. suspects that it will abate considerably over the next few weeks. During their initial interviews Dr X. concentrates on calming Mrs N.L., although he does also complete the first stage of the assessment, during which he examines the extent and nature of Mrs N.L.'s delusions. Delusions do not always render people incompetent; they produce incompetency only if they impinge on the ability to perform a specific task. Dr X. therefore wants to know whether Mrs N.L. is suffering from any delusions with regard to her lawyer, or the proposed legal proceedings – for example, is she hearing voices that tell her not to take her husband to court or that her lawyer is an agent of the Royal Canadian Mounted Police who has been sent to harm her? On speaking with her Dr X. is satisfied that Mrs N.L. is either not suffering from auditory hallucinations or, if she is, they are not impinging on her thoughts about her lawyer or the proposed legal proceedings. Mrs N.L.'s delusions have not deprived her of the ability to instruct counsel.

As Mrs N.L.'s emotional condition stabilizes, the psychiatrist focuses on her ability to retain legal information and to make decisions about her legal affairs. He first reviews with her the information that the lawyer has provided him with, and he asks her to repeat it to him in her own words, a task that she performs quite well. Then they discuss her options – for example, that she can bring the lawsuit or not bring it. She tells him that she wants to bring the lawsuit; her husband treated her wrongly and should make amends to her. She also needs money desperately, and a lawsuit is the only way to get it. Finally, she no longer trusts or loves her husband and does not want to be married to him. The psychiatrist goes over the legal information with her at three separate sessions, and during the latter two she is able to recount the information accurately without prompting; she also repeats the same decision and reasoning about the lawsuit. She clearly understands, and welcomes, the solemnity and finality of legal proceedings. She understands that if she brings a lawsuit she may have to reveal personal matters and be assessed by an unfamiliar psychiatrist; although she does not welcome either possibility she understands that they are the price she must, and is willing to, pay for suing her husband. She is also aware of the degree of trust that she is being asked to repose in her lawyer and has confidence in him; he did not abandon her despite her poor performance at their initial interview, and he has tried to find a way to help her.

At their final session the psychiatrist asks a series of questions that test her ability to exercise judgment. He asks, for example, what she would do if her lawyer told a judge that she did not want to divorce her husband. She answers that she would tell the judge that her lawyer was wrong. He also asks her whether she would withdraw her lawsuit if the lawyer told her that she could not possibly win it. She answers that she would. Her psychiatrist is completely satisfied that she understands what a lawsuit is and can comprehend and make independent decisions on the basis of legal advice, and he prepares a report for the lawyer saying so.

Mrs W.: Testamentary capacity, or competency to make one's will

Mrs W. is a woman in her eighties who has suffered a stroke that has substantially impaired her memory and left her somewhat confused. Her competency fluctuates, and she is much more alert in the morning than she is in the evening. She wishes to change her existing will, disinheriting some of her present beneficiaries and increasing the amount she will leave to others. Her oldest son, who is also the executor of her will, arranges to have her lawyer visit her. The lawyer is not certain that Mrs W. possesses testamentary capacity because she cannot recall the contents of her existing will and because her degree of mental alertness varies. The lawyer asks the medical director of Mrs W.'s nursing home to arrange a competency assessment for her.

Testamentary capacity

A person who possesses testamentary capacity must recognize that a will is a legally binding instrument that provides for the disposition of his or her property after death. In addition the person must recognize all the property that he or she has to dispose of; know the range of potential donors to whom he or she would ordinarily be expected to leave a bequest; and have the ability to relate this legal information to his or her own life and to make independent testamentary decisions.

Mrs W.'s lawyer knows that her will is likely to be contested by the beneficiaries whom she proposes to disinherit. When a will is challenged it is often attacked on two grounds: that the testator lacked testamentary capacity, and that the testator came under undue influence. Although a competency assessment is generally directed to the issue of testamentary capacity, it may also be relevant to the issue of undue influence. This is so for two reasons. The assessment itself will often grant a person an opportunity to speak his or her mind in the absence of anyone who may be attempting to shape it. It may also offer some insight into a person's general ability to formulate and execute his or her own decisions.

Preparing for the assessment

The medical director arranges to have a clinical psychologist (Dr Y.), who has a great deal of experience in assessing the competence of elderly people, visit the nursing home and assess Mrs W.'s competency. He provides Dr Y. with Mrs W.'s medical records, which include a recent psychological test that reveals fairly considerable loss of long- and short-term memory. The records also show that Mrs W.'s hearing and eyesight are quite good, so Dr Y. knows that he will not have difficulty communicating with her. Dr Y. speaks with Mrs W.'s nurses and learns that she is at her best in the morning, so he arranges a morning visit with her. He also speaks with Mrs W.'s son and asks him to inform her in advance of his visit and of the reason for it. Mrs W. asks her son to be present when she meets Dr Y. and he agrees to be.

The initial visit

Dr Y. explains to Mrs W. that he is a psychologist and that he has come because her lawyer has some doubts about her ability to make a new will. He tells Mrs W. that he wants to help her make a new will, but that if she agrees to the assessment he might conclude that she cannot do so. He then describes to her in broad outline the procedures that are part of his standard assessment. It is, he tells her, entirely her decision whether to go ahead with the assessment. Mrs W. consents and Dr Y. explains to her that he prefers to conduct his assessments in private. She agrees to have her son leave the room, and Dr Y. administers the Mental Status Examination to her. His results are very similar to those in her medical records – she has a considerable memory problem, but she is able to assimilate new information and to exercise judgment. By the time she has completed the test Mrs W. is tired, and her speech and concentration are deteriorating rapidly. Dr Y. decides that their future meetings will be no longer than one-half hour in length. Before leaving he asks for and receives Mrs W.'s permission to discuss her affairs with her son, who holds her enduring power of attorney and manages her finances for her.

The psychologist is now certain that the major hurdle Mrs W. will have to overcome is her poor memory. To facilitate his assessment of her memory he asks Mrs W.'s son to prepare a list of Mrs W.'s assets. Although the son is reluctant to participate at all in his mother's will-making (he disagrees with her decision to disinherit some of her relatives) he also recognizes her right to make her own testamentary decisions if she is able to. He therefore prepares the requested list. Dr Y. also asks Mrs W.'s lawyer to provide him with a copy of her existing will and a summary of the changes that she proposes to make to it.

The assessment

At his next visit Dr Y. begins a task-specific assessment. He asks Mrs W. to tell him what a will is; she says that it is her way of deciding who will get her property when she dies. He asks her what an executor does, and she says that an executor must follow her wishes after she dies. He asks her whether a will takes effect immediately or after she dies, and she answers that it takes effect after death. Her ability to recognize all her property is, in fact, not the serious issue that Dr Y. had thought it would likely be. Her principal assets are cash and liquid investments such as stocks and bonds; all that she must understand is the approximate cash value of her estate and the approximate value of each bequest that she proposes to make.

Dr Y. next asks her to name all those whom she might want to consider as potential beneficiaries. She names all the people whom she recognized in her original will. She cannot recall the contents of her existing will but Dr Y. reviews it, bequest by bequest, with her. She recognizes each bequest and is able to explain why she made it. There are a number of bequests that she now wishes to eliminate from her will, and she is able to explain in each case why she wishes to do so; she wishes to reward those who have been faithful to her in her illness and to punish those who have abandoned her. The changes that she tells Dr Y. she wishes to make are the same as the changes that she told her lawyer she wanted to make. The psychologist repeats this exercise with her at each of the three following sessions. Although her alertness and fluency waver, she consistently displays an understanding of what a will is, and identifies the same group of people to disinherit and the same group to reward.

After four half-hour sessions Dr Y. is satisfied that Mrs W. has an adequate grasp of the nature of a will, the extent of her assets, and the range of potential beneficiaries. He is also convinced that her decision to disinherit some beneficiaries is her own independent and reasoned choice. During these sessions he has also probed Mrs W.'s ability to exercise judgment, and he now schedules one final session to complete this aspect of the assessment. During it he asks Mrs W. whether she would change her will again if one of the people whom she proposes to disinherit has a change of heart and begins to visit her regularly. Although she doubts this will happen, she says that she certainly would think about doing so. Dr Y. also discusses the potential consequences of her decision, reminding her that her will might be contested after her death and that a legal dispute of this kind often irrevocably splits a family. She says that she recognizes that this is so, but that those who abandoned her have already split the family beyond repair. As well, she will not allow bad people to bully her into giving them anything. Finally, the psychologist probes her ability to resist pressure. Toward the end of the interview, as she is beginning to tire, he tells her that many people will think that her decision is wrong and selfish and would advise her to reconsider it. She is energized by this challenge and adamantly states that no one has any business telling her what to do.

Dr Y. concludes that Mrs W. is indeed exercising judgment: she is prepared to reconsider her decision in the light of any future changes in circumstances that are relevant to her concerns, and she recognizes and accepts the likely consequences of her behavior. She is clearly capable of formulating independent decisions and of resisting outside influence. Dr Y. concludes that Mrs W. possesses testamentary capacity. He immediately informs Mrs W. of his conclusion, and later prepares a written report for her lawyer. As well, he attends the signing of Mrs W.'s new will to assure himself that she remained competent throughout the entire process of will-making.

Mr P.A.: Competency to grant a power of attorney

Mr P.A. suffers from a progressive dementia; before it was diagnosed he began to spend money recklessly and to behave abusively towards his wife and children. His wife threw him out of their house before she realized that his erratic behavior was caused by his illness. His dementia was diagnosed by a neurologist who suspected that Mr P.A. would soon be unable to make his own financial decisions. The neurologist told Mrs P.A. that people like Mr P.A. often execute an enduring power of attorney but that Mr P.A. might not have the mental capacity to do so. Mrs P.A. agreed that she would consult a lawyer; the neurologist agreed to arrange for a competency assessment. The neurologist referred Mr P.A. to a psychiatrist (Dr Z.), but Mrs P.A. never made an appointment for her husband. Mrs P.A.'s strong and conflicting emotions over her husband's illness left her in a state of emotional paralysis. However, Mr P.A.'s condition has continued to worsen; his memory lapses are more frequent, his attention span shorter, and his speech is increasingly disjointed and incoherent. Mrs P.A. is exhausted from the strain of caring for him twenty-four hours a day (he sleeps very little, often pacing the house for much of the night). As well, she has spent most of the money from their joint savings account, and she must sell some of her husband's real property to raise money. Ultimately circumstances force Mrs P.A. to come to terms with the need to establish some arrangement for ongoing financial substitute decision making on her husband's behalf. She arranges an appointment with a lawyer and with a psychiatrist.

The lawyer

Mrs P.A. takes Mr P.A. to meet with a lawyer, Ms L. Mrs P.A. tells Ms L. about Mr. P.A.'s condition and about his earlier financial misdeeds; she asks Ms L. to prepare an enduring power of attorney that will allow her to sell some of her husband's real property. Mr P.A. says nothing and, to Ms L., does not appear to be following the conversation. Ms L. explains that she can prepare an enduring power of attorney for Mr P.A. only if he wants her to and is mentally competent to give her instructions. She then asks Mrs P.A. to leave her alone with Mr P.A. and engages in a short conversation with him.

Mr P.A. will not spontaneously converse with Ms L., but he will reply to her questions. He appears to understand that she is a lawyer. When Ms L. asks Mr P.A. whether he knows what a power of attorney is, he says that it lets someone 'handle things' for him. When asked whether an agent can do what she wants or must take orders from him, he says that she must take orders from him. When asked whether he would like his wife to be his agent, he says yes. Mr P.A. does appear to grasp the concept of agency, but further questioning reveals that he cannot remember what property he has, and he clearly does not understand what an *enduring* power of attorney is. As well, he gives Ms L. inconsistent instructions. When asked if he wants his wife to sell his property he says yes, but when asked if he does not want her to sell his property he also says yes.

Ms L. suspects that Mr P.A. is merely passively acquiescing to any suggestions that are put to him and is not competent to execute an enduring power of attorney. She tells Mr P.A. that she cannot prepare a power of attorney for him unless he first sees a psychiatrist, and he agrees to do so. Although Ms L. doubts his ability to consent to an assessment she is prepared to go forward on the assumption that he can. The problem, of course, is that only the assessment will tell her whether he is or is not competent, and if he is presumed to be incompetent to consent no assessment may be performed. She then calls Mrs P.A. back into the room and explains that she wants Mr P.A. to visit a psychiatrist. Mrs P.A. tells her that she has already arranged a visit with Dr Z., whom Ms L. agrees to phone.

The psychiatric assessment

Ms L. calls Dr Z. and tells her that she thinks Mr P.A. is incompetent to execute an enduring power of attorney. She explains to Dr Z. why she has drawn this conclusion, and she also outlines the legal test for competency to execute an enduring power of attorney. Dr Z. tells Ms L. that she has, in effect, conducted an informal assessment of competency, on the strength of which Dr Z. concludes that there is ample necessity for a formal competency assessment. Having received a detailed letter of referral from Mr P.A.'s neurologist, Dr Z. also knows about Mr P.A.'s earlier uncontrolled spending and also that Mr P.A.'s memory is impaired. Dr Z. therefore calls Mrs P.A. She asks Mrs P.A. to prepare a list of her husband's property and to bring it with her when he comes for his assessment.

At their meeting Dr Z. makes Mr P.A. comfortable and then obtains his consent to the assessment. Dr Z., like Ms L., is reluctant to deny a person an assessment on the basis of his lack of ability to consent to it, for by doing so she might deprive a competent person of the opportunity to make his own decisions. She administers a Mental Status Examination. It shows that Mr P.A.'s memory loss is extreme and that his near-term memory is affected more than his long-term memory, although both are significantly impaired; thus Mr P.A. is able to remember from his past experience what a power of attorney is, but he has never heard before of an enduring power of attorney and now cannot learn what one is. The test also shows that Mr P.A.'s judgment is substantially impaired. When the doctor goes through the list of his assets with Mr P.A. he recognizes only half the items on it. At times he forgets what question he has been asked before he can answer it. He says that he wants his wife to be his agent and do what she wants with his property, but a few minutes later says that he will not allow anyone to sell any of his property. Mr P.A. refuses to acknowledge that he spent money profligately or unwisely, and (five minutes after saying that he wants his wife to be his agent) denies that he ever wanted any help with his financial affairs.

By now, Dr Z. suspects that Mr P.A. is incapable of making an independent choice. She presents him with a series of options, naming, one at a time, three different people whom he might want to appoint as his attorney. The three are Mr P.A.'s wife, his neurologist, and Dr Z.'s secretary. In each case Mr P.A. assents to Dr Z.'s suggestion that he appoint the named person as his attorney. Dr Z. concludes that the combination of Mr P.A.'s memory disabilities and inability to exercise judgment have not only deprived him of the ability to instruct a lawyer, but have probably rendered him incompetent to make most of his own decisions. Still, there is a slim chance that Mr P.A. will perform better if tested in his own home rather than in her office, so she arranges a home visit. Mr P.A. is the same at home as he was in her office; his disease has rendered Mr P.A. extremely incompetent.

The psychiatrist reports to Ms L., who informs Mr and Mrs P.A. that she cannot prepare an enduring power of attorney for him. Ms L. knows that Mrs P.A. now has no choice but to apply to become Mr P.A.'s guardian. Having acted as Mr P.A.'s lawyer, Ms L. would be in a position of conflict of interest if she now acted as Mrs P.A.'s lawyer on an application to become his guardian. She refers Mrs P.A. to another lawyer. When Mrs P.A. sees this new lawyer and relates her story, she is told that she should apply to become Mr P.A.'s guardian and instructs the lawyer to proceed with a guardianship application.

Guidelines for designing plans for substitute decision making

1 In general, self-designed plans for substitute decision making are preferable to imposed ones, if either will supply adequate protection to an incompetent person.

2 Even when competency is not an issue and there is no immediate

reason to fear it will be, prudent people may wish to consider the advantages of preparing a plan for care in case of need.

3 In planning for possible future incompetency, the advice of a knowledgeable health-care practitioner, or lawyer, or both, often is required.

4 In general, the principle of least-restrictive alternative should prevail.

5 A range of relatively informal, inexpensive, and flexible devices exist to help deal with financial incompetence. They include jointly held property and bank accounts, bank powers of attorney, and representative payees. The living trust is a more formal device that can be used for substitute decision making.

6 The enduring or durable power of attorney is probably the most commonly used and flexible device for self-designed substitute decision making. Depending on local laws, powers of attorney may be used in relation to finances and property, or personal decision-making, or both.

7 The making of a will is often the first step leading to a comprehensive plan for substitute decision making.

8 Advance directives allow a person to express his or her wishes about the personal care (and especially the medical treatment) that he or she will receive if he or she becomes incompetent. The living will is an advance directive that applies to care at the end of life.

9 In making living wills, the process of reflection and discussion leading up to them is often as valuable as the resulting document. Open communication between the maker of a living will and the people who are to implement it is usually essential if its provisions are to be followed.

10 Professionals who help others make living wills should document the competency of the maker.

11 There is some risk of abuse in self-designed plans that will be carried out entirely on a private basis. To minimize these risks the person making such a plan should, perhaps with the help of others:

a consider his or her likely future needs, and choose a substitute decider who has the technical skills and personal characteristics to meet them;

b discuss with the chosen substitute his or her desires regarding the kind of care he or she wishes to receive if wholly or partially incompetent;

c consider appointing alternate substitute decision makers in case the chosen one becomes unable or unwilling to act;

d make appropriate resources available to the substitute decision maker, so that the burden of providing care is manageable for both principle and agent;

e consider incorporating safeguards in the plan, so that the substitute decision maker will begin to act only when needed, and then will assume powers that are only as wide as needed for the extent of the incompetency;

f consider incorporating in the plan some form of outside review or scrutiny of the substitute decision maker.

12 A person who is partially incompetent – that is, incapable of choice in one area of life – may still be able and willing to appoint a substitute decision maker and so forestall the need for an imposed arrangement such as guardianship.

13 Even when a partially incompetent person does not require immediate substitute decision making, he or she should be given an opportunity to consider appointing one as a safeguard against future deterioration.

14 An informal or formal assessment of competency is an essential part of planning for the care of a partially incompetent person. The care the person receives should be proportional to the extent of his or her incompetence.

15 Assessors should be prepared to hold an assessment in abeyance while a partially incompetent person seeks advice from a health-care professional, lawyer, or other appropriate source.

16 Assessors should have background knowledge of various informal devices, so that they can explain them to people for whom they may be useful. These include the devices listed in point 5 above, as well as the simple and practical approach of 'working things out' with family and friends.

17 Although assessors should be prepared to suggest that a person appoint a substitute decision maker, and to offer general information about likely options, they must be careful to avoid imposing their views on others. In general, if someone indicates a desire to plan for his or her own substitute decision making, assessors should refer that person to an independent professional for advice.

18 Anyone who advises frail, vulnerable, or partially incompetent people should be careful to avoid exercising undue influence over their decisions, especially with respect to their wills. In particular, advisers should resist letting good intentions become an excuse for pressuring others to do what the advisers think is best or want them to do.

Conclusion

This book began by considering incompetency as it manifests itself in the lives of people who suffer from it and in the lives of their friends and relatives. Many people feel a strong, deeply rooted, desire to help people whose incompetency has made them less able, or unable, to care for themselves. This book depends on, articulates, and serves that desire to care.

But merely having a desire to care is not alone a sufficient basis for delivering the right kind and amount of care. Those who provide care to incompetent people must do so thoughtfully. Before acting, people should carefully identify the needs of an incompetent person, and devise a plan to meet those needs with as little effort on their part and as little deprivation of the incompetent person's liberty as possible. By establishing a clear purpose for intervening in an incompetent person's life, and choosing the best means of doing so, people may gain many concrete advantages. First, they may avoid exhausting their own willingness or ability to continue caring for an incompetent person. Second, they are more likely to elicit and maintain a strong and loving relationship with the person for whom they care. Third, they can minimize the confusion and distress that incompetency brings with it. And, most important, they can have the satisfaction of knowing that the care they provide is a true manifestation of love, concern, and respect for the person who receives it.

The goal of care is to protect people from the consequences of age, infirmity, or disease while compromising their independence as little as is reasonably possible. In technical language this goal is expressed as the principle of the least-restrictive alternative. In human terms the principle is generally fulfilled by providing care that allows people to live the most vigorous, happy, and independent lives they possibly can. People who wish to meet these goals should begin by informally assessing the needs of those for whom they care. The goal of such assessment is to determine whether there is reason to fear (not conclude) that a person is incompetent, and if so in respect of what kinds of activities.

With this information it is possible to decide what action to take. In some cases it may be possible to care for a person adequately without further competency assessment. In other cases an assessment may be required but can be directed toward a positive goal, for example, to determine whether an incompetent person is able to execute a durable power of attorney. Sometimes guardianship may be the only realistic answer to the needs of an incompetent person, but often it is possible to forestall or eliminate the need for it.

If a formal assessment of competency is necessary, the person who receives it, and his or her relatives or friends, are entitled to demand that it be conducted properly. An assessment should not generally be conducted without the consent of the person who receives it. Then the assessment should be task-specific, thorough, and fair.

Assessors should have an adequate knowledge of the legal devices by which people in their locality may voluntarily appoint a substitute decision maker. When performing assessments that may lead to guardianship, assessors should consider the possibility that a partially incompetent person may be able, and willing, to take advantage of such devices. As well, assessors should be aware of their responsibility to safeguard the liberty of those whom they assess. Except in cases involving people who are obviously competent or incompetent, it is reasonable to question the validity of 'one-shot' assessments that involve only a single meeting with the person being assessed.

Whenever possible, partially incompetent people should be encouraged to plan for their own care. The provision of care that accords with the incompetent person's own wishes or instructions is often the most satisfying and fruitful approach to answering his or her needs. There are good reasons to believe this. First, with such care the possibility of friction between giver and recipient is minimized, although not eliminated. Second, it is often difficult for one person to approximate the wishes that an incompetent person would express if he or she were competent to do so; this uncertainty can be gravely troubling, especially when substitute deciders must make decisions regarding the care that an incompetent and dying person is to receive. Finally, to follow someone's own wishes or instructions is often a powerful display of fidelity and respect.

It is particularly important for people who are already partially incompetent, or who are suffering from diseases or conditions that are likely soon to render them incompetent, to choose, appoint, and instruct a substitute decision maker. Moreover, even people who are healthy and vigorous, and who can reasonably expect to continue so for the foreseeable future, may wish to make such a plan. There can be considerable reassurance in providing for one's own care in the event of incompetency, and such planning may also spare relatives and friends considerable effort and frustration. In general, people who wish to plan for the possibility of incompetence will require the assistance of a local health-care provider, or a lawyer, or both. It is essential that people acquaint themselves with their local laws and practices before establishing a plan for substitute decision making on their own behalf or on behalf of another. This book is a only guide to thinking about incompetency, not a self-help book.

Incompetency is not a happy subject, but is an unavoidable one. The reality is that almost everyone is likely to become incompetent at some point in his or her life. The North American population is an aging one and people are living longer lives. With an older population comes an increase in the prevalence of incompetency. Many North Americans will be touched, in one way or another, by mental incompetency and the problems that it creates. They will have no choice but to come to terms with this reality. They may do so by planning for their own care, should they become incompetent, and by providing decent and thoughtful care to others who require it. Those who recognize that they may become incompetent, and face up to this reality in a sober and intelligent way, display mature self-acceptance and self-mastery. Those who display love, respect, and concern for incompetent people enhance their own humanity. Incompetency is a human problem, a proof of human fragility and impermanence. In meeting incompetency with intelligence and dignity, people treat human frailty as an occasion for affirming human strength and goodness.

Index